PSYCHIATRIC DISORDERS IN OLD AGE

SECOND EDITION

Psychiatric Disorders in Old Age

A Handbook for the Clinical Team

TONY WHITEHEAD MB BS MRCPsych DPM

Consultant Psychiatrist, Department of Geriatric Psychiatry, Bevendean Hospital, Brighton

With a Foreword by FELIX POST MD FRCP FRCPsych

Formerly Consultant Psychiatrist, the Bethlem Royal and the Maudsley Hospitals, London

AN HM+M PUBLICATION

Distributed in USA by

Springer Publishing Company

New York

Second Edition 1979
Published by HM+M Publishers Ltd
Milton Road, Aylesbury, Buckinghamshire, England

Distributed by Springer Publishing Company Inc
200 Park Avenue South
New York, New York 10003

ISBN 0-8261-1680-9

Printed in Great Britain
by Maund & Irvine Ltd, Tring, Hertfordshire

Contents

Foreword

As people grow older they become slower in movement and thought. Memory and learning ability decrease. Adjustment to new demands becomes more difficult, and there is, possibly in self-defence, a tendency to withdraw from social participation. All these changes are so slowly progressive and slight that in the great majority of people the shifts in personality functioning due to age cause no trouble to the old persons themselves or to their friends and families.

Unfortunately, the ageing personality is exposed to many psychological and social stresses, of which the most important are loss of spouse, the moving away of children, deaths of relatives and friends, retirement, financial stringency, and poor housing. Even more important, physical illnesses tend to become increasingly frequent, disabling and persistent. Finally, the organ of the mind, the brain, may be attacked by pathological processes of a kind which become increasingly common with rising age. For all these reasons, a sizeable proportion of elderly people suffer from emotional disorders or from the effects of cerebral failure. Severe psychiatric illnesses have been found in some 10 per cent of all people over 65, and this proportion rises to some 60 per cent in those who are afflicted with persistent physical ill health. Minor psychological symptoms are very common even among healthy old people.

Many members of the medical and other "helping" professions have had no training to enable them to recognise major or minor psychiatric conditions, to evaluate their importance in elderly persons, and to guide them towards the appropriate kind of management and (where this is possible) treatment. Services for the aged are unlikely to become effective until these shortcomings have been remedied. Written from experience, Dr Tony Whitehead's presentation of practical situations should succeed in promoting greater awareness of mental problems, and lead towards their more rational management.

FELIX POST

To the American Reader

Since the first edition of *Psychiatric Disorders in Old Age* received such a warm welcome in the United States, we are pleased to present this revised and updated version to our American readers. Although written by a British psychiatrist for British health services personnel, the approaches to the care of the elderly with psychiatric disturbances are equally applicable in this country. The case studies reported involve recent developments in the care of patients whose counterparts may be found in any society in which longevity has been pursued as a desirable objective. In addition, development of means for making people's advanced years useful and enjoyable, as well as healthful, has recently received much attention, and readers will find Dr Whitehead's suggestions both useful and practical. In view of the universality of the conditions and therapies described, the text of the book has not been americanized.

Preface

THE FIRST EDITION of this book came out in 1974 as a practical handbook for geriatricians, psychiatrists, family doctors, students and all members of the team that should be involved in providing a service for old people with psychiatric illness. It was suggested at that time that it was essential to develop the concept of the team, so that everyone who is needed to provide treatment, help and support, could be actively and democratically involved in helping old people. This must include nurses, family doctors, social workers, psychiatrists, occupational therapists, physiotherapists, speech therapists, voluntary workers, home helps, community nurses and a host of other people who play an important role in the care and support of the elderly psychiatric patient.

Since then it has become progressively more obvious how essential it is to develop the team approach. The days are going when the doctor is all-powerful and members of other disciplines are simply his acolytes. Doctors do not have a corner in knowledge and understanding and other workers in the so-called caring services need to be able to contribute as equals, and not servants.

It is doubtful whether any patient with any kind of illness should be treated as if he were suffering from that illness in isolation from all else. Narrow concepts of diagnosis and treatment can have little place in the effective provision of care and support of the elderly. Old people usually have many problems and many pathologies, so the diagnosis needs to include much more than placing a psychiatric label on them. Diagnostic labels have been used in this book because they have a limited role, but the use of a label must never detract from treatment of the individual as an individual, with his own unique problems, anxieties, disabilities and strengths.

An account is given of the kinds of services that should be available to old people; these are minimal services and should not be looked upon as the ideal. It is important that these minimal services be developed as quickly as possible, so that we can move forward to really providing help where it is needed and is most effective, in the patient's home.

There is a lot of despair about the problems created by an ever-increasing population of elderly people. Not only is this despair unwarranted but it can be very destructive. Many good services for the elderly have already been developed in this country and workers in areas where such services do not exist should go to see what is being done, and in turn develop their own services, not necessarily in the same way but along similar lines modified by local needs and conditions.

All may not agree with the opinions expressed here and I should hope this will be the case, since thoughtful disagreement is the essence of progress.

Many people, including patients, have contributed to this book. They are too numerous to acknowledge individually by name, but I should like to take this opportunity to thank them all; they include those patients whose case histories I have used. In the interests of anonymity I have changed their names.

Brighton, 1978 TONY WHITEHEAD

CHAPTER 1

Introduction

ALL SOCIETIES produce their myths, and our society seems to be particularly good at myth production. One generally-believed myth is that ours is a society in which there is no poverty and all citizens are pampered and protected from the whims of fortune by The Welfare State. Over the past thirty years the Establishment has made some effort to help people, as distinct from being more concerned with national status and profit, but large numbers of people still suffer from poverty, poor housing and other degregations. The elderly make up a reasonable proportion of those still deprived.

Another commonly held mythological belief is that there are too many old people around and that their numbers are increasing at such a rate that social catastrophy is almost inevitable. There is, of course, an increasing proportion of old people, and the birth rate is decreasing because fewer unwanted children are being born. A spread in the knowledge of contraception and a slightly more enlightened law on abortion has made sexual joy possible without the dreaded consequences of the unwanted pregnancy and the unwanted child. Because of these happenings some people trapped in sexual inhibition, distorted moral teachings, and generally anti-life attitudes make dismal forecasts for the future. Bemoaning legalised abortions on the one hand they express fears that soon the old will be put down under the guise of euthanasia.

There has been no dramatic increase in life expectancy for the individual, but there is a considerable increase in the number of people who now reach old age. Advances in social organisation and administration, public health and, to a lesser degree, medical techniques, have increased everyone's chance of survival. Efforts to prevent and cure disease have reaped a harvest of elderly people that society now treats as a problem. Unfortunately, there is a tendency throughout society to overvalue the so-called productive adult and look upon people who are no longer allowed to be productive as a nuisance, and more than a nuisance if they are in need of medical help and social support. Certainly, an increase in the proportion of old people in a society must mean that there is an increase of both physical and mental illness and more demands upon the supports that society can provide. This should not mean that these demands cannot be dealt with. In fact it appears that they can be dealt with, provided society wants to deal with them. Aside from the normal consequences of ageing, a number of correctable factors operate in producing disability in the elderly. Compulsory retirement at some magically-decided-upon age can be an important factor in creating disability, particularly psychological disability. To stop work suddenly, cease to be important and find nothing to do all day can be extremely traumatic. Some people welcome retirement as an opportunity to do all the things they had little time for when they were working, but this does not apply to the majority, who may look upon retirement with dread which becomes a reality once the 60th or 65th birthday has passed. Not only does retirement bring loss of status, feelings of uselessness and boredom but to this is added poverty, poor housing, social isolation and everything else that goes with being a member of a deprived group. This deprivation applies to everything from being impatiently disregarded by shopkeepers and local government officials to difficulties in receiving help and treatment when ill. It is rarely difficult to get a 50-year-old man with a coronary thrombosis, an acute abdomen or a fracture admitted to hospital, rapidly treated and equally rapidly rehabilitated and returned to a normal life in the community. If the same man happens to be over 65 admission to hospital may be difficult, if not impossible, and once in hospital there may not be the same feeling of urgency to get him well and back on his feet. There will be concern about how he can be got out of what is so dreadfully described as a 'valuable bed' into some other establishment where he will be out of sight and out of mind.

Society's attitude to the elderly at its worst is illustrated by the statement of a physician who once requested a geriatrician to "get this geriatric grot out of my ward", and the grocer who said to a social worker involved in work with the elderly "Why does a young girl like you waste your time on these old fools, when you could be doing something more useful?". These are extreme views and very many people would strongly object to them, considering, quite rightly, that old people have the same rights as anyone else in our society.

It is sometimes said that families now reject their elderly relatives and instead of caring for them, expect society to do it so that they can be free to live their own lives unencumbered and unconcerned. This view is often expressed by people working in the medical and social services, but it is yet another myth, since the great majority of families do support their elderly relatives with little help from anyone. Workers in the health and social services may get a distorted picture of what happens to old people because they see only those that are apparently rejected and often have little contact with the ones that are being supported by their families.

The fact that the majority of families care for their elderly relatives is not a contradiction of what has been said before, since very many old people have no families, and some are members of families in which there has been lifelong maladjustment and tension, sometimes engendered by the old person throughout his or her life, so that rejection occurs when behaviour or illness ruptures the strained ties.

This group of the isolated and rejected places a major strain upon the medical and social services and is, on the whole, inadequately catered for and, in turn, often rejected by these services. A consequence of this is that not only are the various agencies overloaded but because the strains upon them appear to be due to having to deal with old people, old people who are being supported by their families but need, for one reason or another, medical and social service help, may not be able to find it. This can lead to the family feeling overpowered and helpless, with the result that they may react by finally rejecting the old relative they have supported so well until a crisis occurs.

These are possibly very many ways of approaching the problems that have been briefly described; some of them are fairly obvious and can be broadly divided into long-term and short-term. Long-term action includes the education of the public so that not only can they prepare for their own retirement more effectively than is now possible, but they will be able to deal more successfully with the problems that might arise in old age in themselves or in others.

Coupled with education there should be considerable rethinking about our out-dated economic principles. Technological advance has made it possible for the production of articles to be increased, while the number of people involved in industry can be dramatically decreased. This should result in many more people being available to help and support the disabled, be they young or old. This does not mean that one half of the population would be involved in supporting the other half, but it does mean that there need to be radical changes in education so that children would be prepared either for a future in the various caring and supporting services or would be able to live interesting and useful lives without having to depend on what we now describe as a 'regular job'.

These ideas, even if followed up, would not help the present situation and it is the present situation with which we are now concerned. This book is not a solution to the problem but is an attempt to describe what can be done for a certain group of old people that would not only help and support them but also relieve the strain on the various hospital and social services involved, and on the public.

At the present time a large number of different services and agencies are concerned in providing help, care and treatment for old people. These include the family doctor and hospital service, local authority social service departments, and a variety of voluntary organisations, particularly Age Concern. Large numbers of people are involved with these various organisations and services and spend much time and expertise in helping as many old people as possible. Unfortunately, because there are a multitude of services there is often overlap, duplication, some conflict and little evidence of an overall plan. Individual services may be divided within themselves. For example, the hospital service has geriatric departments and psychiatric departments which cater for old people, while all the other branches deal with a high proportion of elderly patients. The need for co-ordination and close co-operation is obvious, yet in spite of general agreement that this is the case, individual departments may be in conflict with each other. The situation becomes that little bit worse when co-operation between the hospital and the local authority services is considered. Here the added problem of different sources of finance occurs, with the hospital being financed by the central government, while the local authority services are financed, at least in part, from local taxation, i.e. the rates.

The old person who develops a mental illness is in a particularly vulnerable position. Many psychiatric services do not have special facilities for the elderly, while other services are loath to deal with patients who have illnesses they do not understand and may find alarming and threatening. When this is coupled with society's fear of mental illness and the ambivalent attitudes to the elderly in general, the mentally ill old person is in a dismal position. One common result of this situation is that the patient is grudgingly admitted either to a geriatric or a psychiatric bed where she is in danger of remaining for the rest of her life, because the facility is not geared to provide either treatment or effective community support after treatment. Many enter and few leave except as a result of death.

This is one reason why in-patient and residential facilities are so hard-pressed. For example, in 1972 there were 52,000 patients over 65 in hospitals for mental illness, making up almost half the mental hospital in-patient population.

A very good case can be made out for specialisation in the care of the elderly, yet general physicians, surgeons and other specialists are treating an ever increasing proportion of old people. It is not uncommon to find general medical wards in which there are only two or three patients under the age of 65. Since all doctors treat old people, geriatric departments and the few existing specialist psychiatric departments for the elderly are becoming more and more repositories of severely disabled, or apparently severely disabled, old people who everyone else believes are beyond medical help. This can be demoralising, with the possible result that those patients who come into the care of these specialist departments are less likely to be treated hopefully, and those who could get better do not. If medical education was changed sufficiently to give students a realistic and humane idea of their future work, doctors, regardless of their speciality, would expect and be prepared to deal with a majority of old people. They would accept the need to develop services to help the disabled elderly and specialisation in geriatrics would be unnecessary.

At the present time this is not the case and specialisation in treating the old must continue. If this is accepted, specialisation in the psychiatry of old age is also necessary since a large proportion of the psychiatrists conducting psychiatric services have more than sufficient work to do with younger patients, and hence are unlikely to be able to invest the time necessary to develop and operate an effective service for the old. In order adequately to deal with both the old and the young it would be necessary considerably to reduce the individual psychiatrist's work load, and he would either have to produce a mini-service for the elderly or co-operate closely with a number of his colleagues in running a shared service. Either of these could be effective but, remembering present medical and psychiatric education and training, it appears more satisfactory to set up special, separate departments to deal with the old, staffed by people who have voluntarily taken an interest in this group of patients.

A specialist service for the elderly mentally ill can contribute greatly to easing the load on overstrained in-patient and residential facilities, while providing greater help for greater numbers of old people than is possible in the absence of such a service. Specialisation should not mean that others need have no interest in mental illness in the elderly. The more people who know something about the psychiatric diseases that may afflict old people and how the sufferer can be treated and helped, the more likely it is that the individual patient will be recognised as having a mental illness and that things can be done to help and support him without the need for long-term institutional care.

In this book the mental disorders of the old are described with particular reference to treatment and support in the community in the hope that the reader will develop a more hopeful and interested attitude towards old people with mental illness, so contributing to solving one of the major problems of our age.

It must be emphasised that old people in difficulty usually have many troubles, which may include physical disease, or diseases, emotional disturbances, or frank mental illness and a whole variety of social problems. For clarity and easier understanding mental disorders will be described without including too many other symptoms, signs and problems. This must not be taken to mean that patients with mental disorders always present in this easy-to-categorise way. They usually do not, but an understanding of mental disease and its symptoms and signs will make it easier to pick them out, even when the symptoms are muddled up with many other things. People are never 'hearts', 'diabetics', 'depressives' or 'dements': they are always people.

Before considering specific psychiatric syndromes it may be useful to look at three examples of what may happen to old people who become mentally ill, and then examine the part the family and community can play in providing help and support, together with the sort of services that should and can be provided by official agencies and voluntary organisations.

CHAPTER 2

Some Old People

MRS. OLIVE JAMES was admitted to hospital five years ago. She had been widowed 25 years before and had worked as an office cleaner until she was 72. After her husband died of carcinoma of the bronchus she moved from their home to a furnished room: she had tried to get unfurnished accommodation but had been unsuccessful. After giving up work she lost contact with her friends, most of whom had been associated with her work. She tended to spend most of her time in her room, only going out to shop when this was necessary. She started to become forgetful and neglected herself and her room. Restlessness at night disturbed her landlady and then she started to go out at night and was brought back by the police on two occasions. Her landlady, disturbed by this change in behaviour, became worried in case she left the gas on or caused a fire in the house. She did neither of these things, but the landlady was concerned about the possibilities. Her doctor was consulted, who asked for a psychiatric opinion. She was visited at home, welcomed the psychiatrist and offered him a cup of tea, which she never got around to making.

The room was untidy and there was a smell of stale urine; the unmade bed was slightly wet with urine. The old lady was rather untidy, with her stockings twisted and slipping down her legs and a large safety pin holding together the top of her skirt in place of the buttons which should have been there. She said that she felt well and could not understand why the doctor had asked anyone to see her. She could not remember seeing her doctor and believed the last time had been when her husband was dying.

Formal psychiatric examination revealed evidence of poor memory for recent events with a rather patchy recall of more distant events. She showed little concern about her condition and did not appear to mind being seen by a psychiatrist who asked a lot of intimate and, what should have been to her, irrevelant questions.

Her landlady was adamant about not being able to keep her any longer, so the only apparent solution to the situation was her admission to hospital.

Following admission to hospital it was possible to correct her incontinence by habit training and she was accepted by the social service department for placement in an old people's home. Unfortunately, by the time a place was offered she had deteriorated and was no longer looked upon as a suitable candidate.

By now she was in a ward with 45 other old ladies, cared for by very few staff, who did not remain on the ward long enough to develop any sort of relationship with the patients. Attempts were made to provide activity and entertainment, but no-one ever talked to Mrs. James. She never had visitors, and volunteers who visited the ward stopped trying to talk to her because they rarely got any response.

If examined superficially it appeared that she was unaware of her surroundings, or of anything else, but close observation demonstrated the inaccuracy of this assessment. When a real attempt was made to talk to her she would start to respond and obviously had more contact with her surroundings than many would wish to acknowledge or believe. She brightened up when pleasant activities were taking place, such as music, dancing, or visits by local children. For most of the time she was apathetic showing no interest, thinking thoughts that could not be discovered. Her day was spent between a bed with cot sides and a chair that had a little table fixed to it to prevent her falling forward. She died one year ago.

Mrs. Lettie Wood, a widow of 82, attends the day hospital every day from Monday to Friday. She takes part in all the activities provided, dresses reasonably well, appears to be cheerful and has two or three cronies whose table she shares for meals, bingo and rug-making. She lives in a two-roomed flat and has a neighbour who is fond of her.

At the weekends she does not attend the day hospital because it is closed but she is visited by a voluntary worker and her meals are provided by the friendly neighbour.

She has attended the day hospital for five years, having first been referred to the psychiatric service because, over a period of a few weeks, she tended to walk around her flat in the early hours of the morning and, on occasion, to go out shopping at midnight. She also appeared very forgetful to her neighbour and sometimes even failed to recognise her. The neighbour became very concerned and finally persuaded Mrs. Wood's doctor that something might be amiss. He transferred the problem to the psychiatric service and a visit was made by a psychiatrist. He discovered evidence of memory defect, particularly of recent memory. She knew her name, was unsure of her age, her address, the day, the month or the year. She was pleasant and unconcerned, denying that anything was amiss except for some bladder trouble which resulted in little accidents. Her rooms were clean and tidy but this was due in part to the efforts of the neighbour.

In spite of the problem of wandering at night it was decided that day care should be tried. The judicious use of tranquillizers and occupation during the day resulted in her sleeping normally at night. During the first weeks of her attendance she often refused to come to the day hospital when called for by ambulance; this problem was dealt with by a nurse from the day hospital going with the ambulance to pick her up. After three weeks, instead of refusing to come or being unready, she would often be found waiting in the doorway when the ambulance arrived and complained if it was late.

Ten months after attending the day hospital she developed, over one week-end, a fairly severe chest infection, and her family doctor was called by the neighbour on the Sunday evening. He found her to be very confused and delirious and asked for help from the psychiatric service. The emergency team, which consisted of a doctor, two nurses and a social worker, was sent out and found her to be suffering from bronchopneumonia with an associated acute brain syndrome (acute toxic confusional state). Antibiotic treatment was started at once and one of the nurses remained with her for the night. The next morning she was a little better and the neighbour stayed with her for the day. At night a nurse went out again and the following morning she was so much better that it was decided that the day afterwards she would be able to attend the day hospital. That night no nurse was required and the next day she recommenced day hospital attendance. Since then there have been no further problems. Her memory defect has remained unchanged except that she no longer has difficulty in finding her way around the day hospital or its garden, a trouble she had when she first attended.

Mr. James Hall had been an active, socially involved individual all his life and continued to run a small but efficient business until the age of 74, when he had a 'stroke' that affected his right arm and leg and interfered with his speech. He made a fairly rapid recovery, but remained rather confused and continued to have difficulty finding the right word when he spoke.

He had married a girl of approximately his own age when he was in his early twenties and they maintained a close relationship throughout life. Following the stroke he was admitted to a general hospital, but only remained there long enough to become mobilised, when he and his wife agreed that he would be best at home. After he had been at home for approximately one week his family doctor became concerned about his continuing confusion and suggested that he should see a psychiatrist. He and his wife were seen in an out-patient clinic and it was suggested that he would benefit from attending the local day hospital, where it would be possible to assess him further and also provide activities and some speech therapy. The offer was declined but he and his wife both agreed to his having speech therapy. This helped a little, but he continued to have difficulty finding the right word and was still occasionally muddled and confused so that he often got lost when he went out for a walk alone. He continued to attend the psychiatric department as an out-patient and his wife was always keen to discover what further she could do to help him. Because he had got lost on occasions she now accompanied him on all his walks and encouraged him to go for walks with her. She also helped him read the daily paper and persuaded him to take up painting and gardening. Again she helped him considerably with these activities.

Five years after having his stroke he still lives at home with his wife and leads a relatively active existence, in spite of a steady deterioration in his memory and reasoning ability. His wife has every intention of keeping him at home until he dies.

The lessons to be learned from the histories of these three old people are obvious, but taken in isolation nothing is demonstrated or proved. However, very similar comparative histories can be obtained if out-patient and day hospital patients are compared with their contemporaries who have been admitted. These comparisons are difficult to assess since selection must operate with the result that like is not really being compared with like. Mrs. James had a different personality to Mrs. Wood and this may be the reason why one had an unsympathetic landlady and the other a dedicated friend, and Mr. Hall had a loving wife. The only effective way of comparing out-patients and day patients with in-patients is to compare people selected at random. This would be difficult, since circumstance may act against many of those selected for non-institutional care. More important than this practical difficulty would be the complete inhumanity of the whole exercise.

Falling back on impressions, it does appear that when an effective day hospital is provided, with the necessary associated community services, very many old people can be supported successfully in the community who would otherwise have ended their days in some form of institution. It can of course be claimed that patients can be as happy and as contented in institutions as in the community, but this claim is very hard to substantiate. Patients in well-staffed active anti-institutional residential facilities still appear different from those supported in the community. They appear to be less happy and less alert and considerable effort must continually be expended to prevent them slipping into the zombie-like state of the institutionalised human being.

Most in-patient facilities and residential homes are not well-staffed, and it appears unlikely that they will be in the foreseeable future. It can only be destructive to the individual to remove her from society and place her in a situation in which only minimal care and rehabilitation are possible. It may salve society's conscience to place someone who is failing to cope in the community in an institution, with a phantasy aura of effective care, but this is of little benefit to the individual whose life may be turned into half a life.

The history of the elder of the old ladies illustrates the need for a complex of community services associated with day hospital provision. Mrs. Wood was visited by a volunteer at the weekends, and when she became physically ill an emergency team was available to deal with her illness without admitting her to hospital. It can be claimed that her admission to hospital because of her bronchopneumonia is better than treatment at home and cannot be harmful; treatment in hospital may be more effective but the dangers of admission must never be overlooked. Admission to hospital while in a toxic confusional state can result in the confusion continuing after the underlying cause has been dealt with. Removed from the familiar environment and then coming back to reality in a strange and foreign place can be both traumatic and inhibiting to the re-establishment of the patient's tenous contacts with reality. Not only may the patient be disturbed by the experience, but following admission to hospital her place in the community can rapidly disappear: friends and relatives who happily provided support may be loath to give this support back once it has been suspended, and new uses can be found for accommodation in the patient's absence and fears are resurrected to create barriers to discharge. This is the reasoning behind providing effective emergency facilities for old people who become ill or involved in some other crisis situation in the community.

Patients who are as fortunate as Mr. Hall require few, if any, services but such patients are rare, not because loving concerned partners are a rarity but because so often the partner has died, or if alive is disabled in some way. Daughters or sons may try to take on the role of helper and supporter, but the interpersonal relationships are different and they do have their own lives to live. It is right that society should provide the help and support that old people in trouble need and deserve.

Failure to provide day hospital, day centre and other community services, including emergency teams, will result in more and more old people being admitted to hospitals or other residential accommodation with overcrowding, deterioration in care and increasing misery to the individual patients. Developments along these lines are likely to lead to the situation mentioned in the preface with society demanding legalised euthanasia. Society, having mistakenly provided the wrong answer to the problem of its increasing elderly population will want to correct the mistake by killing off the victims of that mistake.

CHAPTER 3

Family, Friends and the Public

IT IS NOT PRACTICABLE to examine and discuss mental disorders or any other type of illness without first looking at people as members of a family and of a community. This would appear to be a statement of the obvious, yet it is easy to forget that a disturbed old lady, living alone, is also a individual with a past and a present, who may have relatives, friends and other people who are significant to her and directly, or indirectly, affect her thoughts, behaviour, and ideas for the future.

Patients are people who have relatives, friends, enemies and many other people who may like them, dislike them, be dependent upon them, or on whom they may depend. It is well known and accepted that a patient cannot be treated in isolation, but needs to be treated as part of a family group and community. Unfortunately, this knowledge and understanding does not mean that patients are not treated in isolation, because it is easier and less traumatic to deal with one individual and his disease. If it is obvious that a young person with a physical illness needs to be treated as part of a family and community, it should be even more obvious that an old person with a mental illness also requires this approach. Old people living in the community are often very dependent on a variety of supports, some overt and others hidden. Not only are family and friends important, but milkmen, postmen, shopkeepers, the boy who brings the paper, the coalman, the representative of the Gas Board or the Electricity Board, the old gentleman who lives across the road and many others may, consciously or unconsciously, provide a web of support, interest and reason for living that if it is destroyed or interfered with can result in disaster. Old people may complain of loneliness, when in fact they have many contacts with other people. When they say they are lonely, they do not necessarily mean that they are isolated from other people, but they do mean that they are isolated from people who are significant to them. These significant people may be relatives, old friends, or members of the groups previously mentioned. A lady living alone may not feel lonely because of these significant contacts, yet can complain bitterly of loneliness if admitted to an institution in which she is in close contact with a large number of people.

Since the old person who becomes a patient is so dependent on these community contacts and may in fact have become ill because of some disturbance in the network of physical and emotional support, effective treatment is only possible if the family and community are involved. Involvement can be particularly difficult if the patient develops a mental illness.

Fear of madness

Most people are afraid of mental illness, both as something that may happen to them, and to others. The public and professionals not involved in the mental health field have strange concepts of mental illness and disturbing fantasies that are far removed from reality. To many, the concept of madness is Mr. Rochester's wife locked away upstairs, with staring eyes, streaming hair and a frightening voice. Fantasy production is not diminished by films, television plays, lurid newspaper reports and popular fiction. Uninformed first-hand experience of someone with a mental illness does not necessarily dissipate these fantasies. The sufferer from a mental illness may behave in rather a wild manner, confirming every hidden and overt fear, but this is very rare and, much more commonly, the patient looks and behaves like someone in distress, harmless and looking for help. This type of behaviour does not alter the fantasy because, expecting madness, it will be found in the expression of a delusional belief, anger, restlessness and many other facets of behaviour that would be looked upon at most as irritating if it was understood that the individual involved was 'normal'. Expecting someone to behave in a mad manner can itself produce behaviour that is interpreted as madness. If you are treated as someone who is strange, and possibly dangerous, it is not surprising that you may react in a manner that confirms these fears. The patient who has successfully recovered from a depressive illness may quite reasonably become angry because of some situation in his domestic environment. This anger would be understood and accepted if there was no previous history of mental illness but, having been treated for depression, it is looked upon as evidence of further mental disturbance and quite often leads to a request for urgent admission to hospital to protect society.

Public standards of normality are extremely variable. An attendant in an old people's home may accept as normal her husband's anger over a peccadillo that she may have committed, yet claim an old lady is going out of her mind if she becomes angry for a similar reason. The old appear to be particularly vulnerable to these distorted concepts of normality. The staff of institutions for the elderly, including psychiatric hospitals, sometimes appear to expect blind obedience, complete emotional control and the acceptance of a passive, furniture-like role. A few relatives also have these attitudes, while neighbours can become very worried by behaviour in an old person that would not excite comment if she was young or middle-aged. If you are young and cannot sleep at night, getting up and making a cup of tea is reasonable behaviour, but if you are old it may be viewed as evidence of 'going senile'.

It must not be assumed from what has been said that the majority of old people who behave abnormally or develop psychiatric symptoms are rejected by their family and friends because they are looked upon as mad and dangerous. In fact, the majority of elderly people with psychiatric symptoms are supported and helped without the intervention of psychiatry. It does mean that mental illness in the elderly, like mental illness in any age group, can generate considerable anxiety, which may result in family and community tensions that will act against any help and treatment provided by psychiatric and geriatric services which are not concerned with the family, neighbours and friends of their patients. This problem will be considered in more detail later, but first a relatively rare but important manifestation of some people's attitude to mental disease will be described.

The gaslight phenomenon

In 1939, Patrick Hamilton published a play entitled 'Gaslight'. Its theme was a husband's plot to get rid of his wife by driving her insane. In 1969, in collaboration with Dr. Russell Barton, I published in *The Lancet* a paper entitled 'The Gaslight Phenomenon' which described real-life plots to get some people wrongly admitted to psychiatric hospitals. All the cases described were definite fraudulent attempts to get rid of an unwanted partner, or in one case, an unwanted resident of an old people's home. The latter was the only example of an elderly victim quoted, but further investigation revealed that the elderly are at risk of being wrongly labelled as mentally ill and taken to hospital, sometimes because of straightforward plots but more commonly as victims of a combination of circumstances.

The old lady quoted in the original paper was a resident of an old people's home and had come in conflict with the matron. She was referred as a case for admission to the local psychiatric unit because of faecal incontinence and agitation. Careful enquiry revealed that the faecal incontinence had been engineered by the matron, who plied the old lady with excessive amounts of laxative. Her agitation appeared to be a direct product of the matron's attitude and actions. Her transfer to another home solved the problem for the patient and the matron without the patient being labelled as mad or the conflict being perpetuated. Working through their differences was not considered practicable and the patient was very keen to move to the other home where she settled quickly and became happy and problem-free.

There are many variations of the gaslight phenomenon that may affect the elderly. Perhaps the best known is where the wrong partner in a marriage or relationship is considered to be mentally ill. A wife suffering from schizophrenia may complain of the odd behaviour of her husband, and it is possible to accept her story when it is found that the husband is emotionally disturbed. I once saw an elderly gentleman whose wife claimed that he had become very 'paranoid', accusing her of following him everywhere he went and spying on all his activities. She also said that he sometimes laughed strangely and talked to himself. The man was rather anxious and depressed, and welcomed the suggestion that he be admitted to hospital. Careful enquiry from the patient, his wife, and a social worker who knew the family revealed that in fact the wife did follow him everywhere and frequently spied upon him to the extent that she would hide in an empty house opposite an inn that he frequented. It finally became clear that the wife was in fact suffering from paraphrenia, spying upon the husband because she believed that he was involved in a complicated plot against her. His mild depressive and anxiety symptoms were fairly easily explainable on the grounds of his wife's changed behaviour. They had been a devoted couple until she became ill, and treatment of her illness resulted in their returning successfully to a normal life together.

Sometimes a patient may develop a psychiatric illness which quickly responds to medication, but later relapses, and it is found that the relative or friend who was supervising treatment has actively discontinued it because of a desire to get the patient admitted to hospital. Sometimes day hospital support is purposefully disrupted by relatives for the same reason. They may claim that it is difficult to get the old person up in time for the ambulance to take her to the day hospital, or they may incorrectly complain that the patient is restless at night; they may inform the staff that the patient is unfit to come, or is afraid to come, or does not like coming. These can be true statements but occasionally they are not, and the person concerned either truly believes the patient would be better treated in hospital or wants her away for a whole variety of reasons. It is ill-advised to make moral judgments in these cases, since few angelic old people are rejected by evil relatives. Conflicts are complex and should be considered dispassionately, with the hope of finding a solution: in some cases this may be admission to hospital, or the provision of some type of accommodation away from the family.

Professional workers, including some family doctors and social workers, may rightly or wrongly decide that an old person should not be supported in the community, and because of this they can consciously, and occasionally unconsciously, sabotage attempts at community support. The support of an old person with a psychiatric illness in the community can be extremely difficult, and because there are difficulties, sabotage is remarkably easy. Exaggeration of the patient's living conditions, making much about being called out at night, and apathy in arranging such supportive services as a home help, or meals on wheels, can all result in the patient being admitted to hospital unnecessarily, where because of the trauma of leaving home, her condition can deteriorate with an end-result that leaves little doubt as to where she should have been treated, but could not be treated because of the obstructive manoeuvres of those who should have been involved in providing support.

The gaslight phenomenon and its variations do occur, and it is important that everyone working in the spheres of geriatrics and psychiatry should be aware of these possibilities. Being aware does not necessarily result in an old person being kept out of hospital, since admission may be the only immediate solution in the face of rejection by those who should have been providing support.

Sometimes rejection can be honest and straightforward. I once treated an old man with an acute toxic confusional state whose wife said, once he had been admitted to hospital, that she had no intention of ever taking him back since he had been a drunkard and womaniser all his life and she had waited 40 years for an opportunity to be rid of him. Another family said they would have nothing more to do with their mother after she had been admitted to hospital following a suicide attempt. Apparently she had been domineering and cruel towards them throughout their whole lives, but they had dutifully rallied round to support her in old age until an opportunity arose for them to escape without leaving her uncared for.

It is usually very difficult to help patients and families that have such disturbed relationships as those in which plots and manoeuvres are used to get rid of the ill or claimed-to-be-ill relative. Fortunately, these families are uncommon.

The great majority of families who find themselves with a mentally ill member do not try to have that member put away at all costs. However, families will have anxieties and fantasies which can produce a whole range of problems. Methods of counteracting these anxieties and fantasy-produced worries will be considered later, but first it may be useful to briefly describe the methods by which a mentally ill individual may be admitted to hospital. This must not be taken to mean that admission to hospital is all important: in fact, the majority of people who become mentally ill can be successfully treated and helped without having to admit them, but some have to be admitted and occasionally this has to be done against their wishes.

Admission to hospital

When an individual becomes mentally ill, or is discovered for the first time to be mentally ill, it is very tempting to consider admission to hospital as a solution to the problem. It may be a quick solution as far as the professional is concerned, but is rarely any sort of solution to the patient's problem. It will continue to be emphasised throughout this book that most mentally ill individuals can be successfully helped and treated in the community. Sometimes admission to hospital is necessary and when it is, it is usually possible to admit the patient informally. An informal admission has a specific meaning as far as mental health legislation is concerned. Prior to the Mental Health Act of 1959, mentally ill individuals were admitted to hospital either compulsorily, or as voluntary patients. Voluntary patients had to sign a form saying they wished to enter the hospital and had to give three days notice before they could leave. The Mental Health Act of 1959 changed this and the intention of the Act was that the majority of mentally ill individuals would be admitted to hospital informally. This was not the same as being a voluntary patient but meant that individuals would be admitted in the same way as someone suffering from a physical disease is admitted to a general hospital. Thus, the patient does not have to sign a form expressing his wish to enter the hospital and in fact can be admitted to hospital without expressing any wish to be admitted. For example, an unconscious patient can be admitted to a psychiatric hospital. However, if the patient specifically says that he does not want to go into hospital he cannot then be admitted informally, and can only be admitted if there are grounds for using compulsion. The informal patient once in hospital is free to leave at any time, unless again there are grounds for compulsory detention.

There are a number of ways of compulsorily admitting someone to hospital.

Emergency admission for observation (section 29)

Section 29 of the Mental Health Act empowers a doctor to admit compulsorily a mentally ill individual to hospital for a period not exceeding three days. For this to happen an application has to be made by either the nearest relative or a social worker recognised under the Mental Health Act, and the application must be supported by a medical recommendation, usually given by the patient's family doctor.

This Section of the Act should only be used when urgent admission to hospital is necessary and it is not possible to get a second medical opinion. There must be good reason to suspect that the patient is either a danger to herself or a danger to others, and social convenience is never a legitimate reason for using compulsion. It should also be remembered that completing the necessary forms does not get the patient into hospital. The patient has to be accepted by the hospital and the hospital can refuse to admit a patient in spite of the appropriate forms being completed.

Admission for observation (section 25)

Section 25 of the Act makes it possible for a patient to be admitted to hospital and there detained for a period not exceeding 28 days. An application for admission must be made by either the nearest relative of the patient, or a social worker approved under the Act, and supported by two medical recommendations which have to be written on a special form. One doctor will usually be the patient's family doctor, and the other doctor must be recognised as having a special knowledge of psychiatry, preferably the consultant psychiatrist who will be responsible for the patient's care in hospital. Again, there should be good grounds for believing that the patient is a danger to herself, or to others.

Admission for treatment (section 26)

This Section of the Act enables a patient to be admitted to hospital and there detained for a period of up to one year. Again, the application can be made either by the patient's nearest relative, or by a social worker, but a social worker cannot make the application if the nearest relative objects. If the nearest relative objects the patient cannot be admitted to hospital, but in certain circumstances it is possible to apply to the County Court to have another person appointed as the nearest relative. As in the case of Section 25 there must be two medical recommendations, one preferably by the patient's family doctor and the other by a doctor with a special knowledge of psychiatry. In the case of Section 26, both doctors must state their reasons for considering the individual mentally ill and why admission has to be under compulsion.

Patients detained under Section 26 of the Act can have the detention order renewed yearly, so in theory may be detained in hospital indefinitely.

Patients admitted compulsorily to hospital under Section 29, Section 25 and Section 26, can be discharged from hospital at any time if this is considered advisable by the consultant psychiatrist responsible for their care. A patient detained under Section 26 may apply to a Mental Health Review Tribunal, who may order his release.

Other methods of being compulsorily admitted to hospital include admission under Section 136, which empowers a police officer to remove to a place of safety a person found in a place to which the public have access, who appears to be suffering from a mental disorder and is in need of control. The patient can then be detained for a period of not exceeding 72 hours. Here there is no need for a medical recommendation. This form of compulsory admission is generally disliked and is rarely used, except in certain black-spots in the country, including Metropolitan London. Patients can also be admitted compulsorily from Court if they have committed an offence and are found to be mentally ill. Section 60 of the Act can be used here and is virtually the same as Section 26. However, Section 65 of the Act makes it possible for someone admitted under Section 60 to have a restriction placed upon his or her discharge by the Judge, so that release is only possible if approval is obtained from the responsible Minister of State, here the Home Secretary.

The compulsory admission of a patient to hospital is a serious and potentially very traumatic action. Compulsion should never be used unless there is a clear and obvious danger to the patient or to others. It should never be used for convenience, or because the patient is being a nuisance to others. Experience has shown that a great majority of patients can be successfully treated without using compulsion. In one unit for the elderly mentally ill, an examination of the use of compulsion over a period of five years revealed that out of an average of 300 admissions per year only 4 to 5 per year were under compulsion.

Since most patients should be and are treated in the community, the attitudes of relatives, friends, and the general public are all important. Not only must relatives and friends be involved in treatment in or out of hospital, but since treatment is likely to occur in the community it is essential that the public in general and neighbours, friends and family in particular, have some understanding of what mental illness is all about. This can be dealt with at two interacting levels.

Public education

For the past few years many efforts have been made to improve the public's knowledge of mental function and mental illness. Articles are written, television programmes are put out almost weekly, many books have been published and psychiatric hospitals have opened their doors so that anyone who is interested can look inside. It is likely that these attempts to educate the public will continue and intensify, but quick results should not be expected. Well-established misconceptions fed by fantasies are hard to correct. Education should, of course, start in childhood and it is odd that it is still rare for children to be taught even simple human physiology and psychology. Perhaps the present faltering attempts to correct this traditional omission will lead to greater and more consistent efforts to teach people a little about themselves at an early stage in their development. The combination of sensible education programmes that place significance on teaching about the human body and its functions, coupled with the present attempts at informing the adult population, will in time not only help the individual to deal more successfully with his fears and fantasies of madness, but make everyone more understanding, sympathetic and helpful in his dealings with those of his fellows who suffer from a mental illness.

It may be said that these pious hopes are all very well but how does this help the psychiatric team to deal with their everyday problems. Firstly, the team members involved in the treatment of patients should invest a little of their energy in trying to improve society's knowledge of illness in all its manifestations. Secondly, every member involved in the psychiatric service, and this includes services for the elderly mentally ill, should as a normal part of his job ensure that some educative programmes are organised. These can range from formal public lectures and talks to various groups in the community, to opening up the hospital or unit to the public so that it ceases to be a place hidden away, out of sight and out of mind, and really becomes a normal part of the community. The latter can be done by encouraging volunteers to help in the wards and departments, allowing free access at all times to relatives and friends, and in every way possible encouraging the community to become involved in what is going on. There is a great untapped source of interested people who can contribute considerable help for our inadequate geriatric and psychiatric services as volunteers. Some hospitals have full-time organisers of volunteers, and their work has shown clearly the existence of this great pool of potential helpers. The introduction of volunteers into hospitals is not a simple task since the professionals at first may be nervous and sometimes rejecting, while the volunteers are even more nervous and hence more likely to take offence. The competent organiser of volunteers must be able to overcome these difficulties and at the same time ensure that the volunteer is matched with the job and is allowed to do the chosen job with the minimum of interference.

A lot of lip service is paid to the concept that the hospital must cease to be remote and inward-looking, and become community-orientated. Unfortunately, the majority of hospitals remain places apart from the community. Some attempts are made to go out into the community, including schemes that allow hospital nurses to treat their discharged patients outside the hospital. These schemes need to be encouraged and considerably extended, with the ultimate goal a situation in which there is no line drawn between patients inside and outside hospital. Steps towards this situation can be taken at once by allowing the unit's nurses to become involved in the care of the patient in the community. Parallel with this, volunteers should become more involved with individual patients and less tied to the hospital on the one hand or the community on the other. If an elderly lady is being visited regularly by a volunteer and is then admitted to hospital, the volunteer should be helped and encouraged to follow the patient to hospital to contribute in whatever way possible to her wellbeing while she is there.

Relatives and friends

In spite of what may or may not be done to improve public knowledge and involve the public in medical and psychiatric services, relatives and friends can, and should, be helped and encouraged to become involved in the treatment and support of their sick member. It has been said before but warrants repetition, that most patients have relatives and friends who are interested and concerned. Some emphasis has been placed on problem families in this chapter. This was done to expose the possible traps that may catch the unsuspecting, and since these traps may result in an individual losing his or her liberty, it was considered worthwhile, even though there was a danger of perpetuating the erroneous belief that many families are rotten.

When assessing and treating a patient, relatives and friends who have been involved with the patient must be welcomed and encouraged to remain involved. This means that their help should be sought at the beginning of treatment and that they are informed as clearly as possible of what is wrong and what it is hoped to achieve. Continued involvement and discussion usually means that the patient's chance of remaining in or returning to the community and surviving there is considerably enhanced. This type of involvement has its dangers. I have known doctors who appeared to specialize in spreading feelings of hopelessness in everyone involved with the patient. If the diagnosis was possibly that of chronic brain syndrome, the relatives would be told that nothing could be done and that the course would be progressively downhill. A common result of receiving this information is a preoccupation with keeping or getting the patient into some type of long-stay institution. Having once established this attitude but later discovering that the initial diagnosis is incorrect and the patient is in fact suffering from a correctable illness, it may be impossible to convince the relatives that this is the case and the patient can return to the community. Even when the diagnosis is correct, offering a little hope is much better than a perhaps correct blackness. Relatives of patients with chronic brain sydrome should not be deceived but should be told that it is possible to help the patient make the most of the abilities he may have retained, and that it is important to have a hopeful attitude if this is to be achieved. A well-known cardiologist used to say that no patient should be the worse for seeing a doctor: the same applies to relatives and the patient's friends.

At the present time very little is done to encourage relatives actively to help with the care of patients in hospital. Some relatives are allowed to do this, but it is usually because of their insistence and not the result of being encouraged by the hospital staff. The staff should in fact persuade and encourage relatives and friends to help, since it both augments the hospital service to the patient, and keeps the patient in the family.

Regular relatives' conferences can play an important part in any unit's service to the patient and public. These are meetings to which all relatives, friends or other interested people are invited and can meet staff members informally. The meeting should be organised in such a way that information is provided by lecture, discussion and demonstration, while perhaps more importantly, an opportunity is provided for the free exchange of views and discussion of problems between all who attend. These discussions allow relatives to compare their problems, exchange ideas on how they have solved them, and give to and receive information from staff members. The exposure of staff to relatives' conferences widens their horizons, helps to correct their misconceptions and gives them greater understanding and sympathy with the patient and his family's difficulties, anxieties and fears. Experience of relatives' conferences has shown that even when a small number of relatives attends, the return in knowledge and the encouragement of greater understanding is well worth the time spent in their organisation. In one hospital regular relatives' conferences produced a number of new ideas that when acted upon proved successful, while the public became more interested in what was happening at the hospital. Out of the meetings, schemes were evolved for raising money to improve the hospital's facilities for patients, and relatives started working in the hospital on a voluntary basis.

Sometimes relatives and concerned friends can be difficult and demanding, which can lead to staff setting up barriers that benefit no-one, least of all the patient. It should be remembered that hospitals can be frightening places. When the patient has a frightening mental illness, those that are concerned about the patient may react by becoming aggressive, querulous and suspicious. The reaction to this should not be anger and rejection, but an effort to instil understanding and tolerance. A pleasant, kindly word usually calms anxiety and counteracts hostility.

CHAPTER 4

Facilities and the Psychiatric Team

THE MAJORITY of old people who are in need of help and support get it from relatives, friends and neighbours and it is only a minority who have to depend upon official and voluntary services. This is as it should be, except when the old person is either inadequately supported by relatives and friends, or has become an intolerable burden upon these people. Official and voluntary services should and must be concerned with providing expert help when it is needed, and ensuring there is support when normal support is absent, inadequate, or over-stressed.

In this chapter consideration will be given to the role of the hospital service in giving help and treatment for old people with psychiatric symptoms. In the past, hospitals tended to confine their activities to providing in-patient accommodation and out-patient advice. This institutional approach still prevails to some degree, but at last there has been a movement towards providing help and treatment where it should be provided, in the community. Hospital staff are now becoming concerned about getting away from the institution. It has also been realised for some time that a number of different people from different disciplines are involved in providing help. The idea that the all-powerful doctor, helped by some subservient nurses can provide all that is needed to treat a patient is now truly dead, and the concept of the multi-disciplinary therapeutic team is evolving and sometimes becoming a reality.

Some doctors still look upon treatment narrowly as something that is done for, or to, the patient that will make him better. This concept of treatment encompasses such things as operations, manipulations, the prescribing of injections, tablets, medicines and ointments, organising physiotherapy, radiotherapy and other technical wonders, but rarely involves much as far as the patient is concerned except his willing acceptance of orders. If the patient is fortunate, other things may be done for him and, on rare occasions, he may be involved in doing things for himself. These accessories can include occupational therapy, participation in recreational activities and even an occasional opportunity to discuss his problems with a social worker. On the whole, psychiatric services are a little better than this and some are much better, yet the elderly patient, even when treated in a progressive, psychiatric milieu, may be dealt with in the same way as the majority of patients in a medical or surgical department.

The treatment of all patients, regardless of their diagnostic label, should involve much more than the mechanical manoeuvres that have been described. Treatment is not something that doctors and nurses do for patients, but involves the total environment in which the patient lives.

Some doctors say that they cannot concern themselves with so-called administrative problems and in hospital are unwilling to become involved in discussions about ward decor, bed types and heights, baths, dining facilities and all the other things that can be dismissed as either nursing or administrative problems. The quaint idea that the treatment and help of patients can be divided up into neat divisions such as clinical and administrative is obviously nonsense. Ill-conceived bed design can be a factor in producing incontinence, poor decor can destroy both staff and patient morale and petty administrative restrictions can do more harm to a patient than any good achieved by prescribing the correct medication.

The treatment of all patients, not least the elderly and the mentally ill, involves attention to everything that is done for them or with them and most important of all, is dependant on the attitudes of those involved in their treatment, care and support. If these people lack sympathy and understanding and fail to deal with the patient as an adult who has dignity and the right to have some say in what goes on about him, no treatment can be really effective. The whole therapeutic regime, be it in the community or the hospital, must be designed to support the patient's dignity as well as to cure or relieve any specific diseases from which he might suffer. As far as possible he should be involved in treatment as an active member of the therapeutic team and the therapeutic team needs to consist of as many people who come in contact with the patient as possible. This means that as well as the doctor or doctors, nurses, psychologists, social worker, occupational therapist, physiotherapist and other professional workers, the orderlies, domestics and porters who may be in close contact with the patient should also be and look upon themselves as being active and participating members of the therapeutic team. This involves their freedom to express opinions about treatment on the same footing as other members of the team. The team, including the patient, must develop a regime in which communication is free and all can speak their mind without any fear of repercussions. It needs to be concerned with the organisation and administration of services which include the type, decoration and furnishing of wards, the provision of facilities within and without the hospital and everything else that goes to make up an effective therapeutic force for the benefit of the patient. Again the patient needs to be involved in all these things as an equal member of the team. It may be said that many patients, particularly elderly ones with dementia, cannot participate in this kind of regime. Obviously there are difficulties but this does not mean that attempts should not be made to involve them as much as possible.

It has been emphasised that treatment is everything that is done or happens to the patient and this means that occupation, entertainment and group activities should be looked upon as being as important as any specific treatment when the word is used in the narrow sense. There is a tendency, even in the most progressive psychiatric hospital, to make every effort to do certain things such as provide medication at the right time, give ECT as necessary, but not invest so much energy in ensuring that other activities take place. Staff become very worried if specific treatments are not given but not so worried if an afternoon of occupation or entertainment does not take place. This is wrong, since the same emphasis should be placed on all facets of treatment and all facets of treatment should be provided.

The team approach

The large number of different services and people involved in providing treatment, help and support for old people with psychiatric illness prohibits them all coming together and forming a genuine team. A therapeutic team, of necessity, must consist of a nucleus of key workers who function closely together, but also relate almost as closely to all the important people who are or should be helping. The nuclear team would normally be made up of representatives of the following disciplines: social work; nursing; psychology; medicine, occupational therapy and physiotherapy and administration, with one or two psychologists, a consultant psychiatrist, two or thre junior doctors, and ideally a consultant geriatric physician with his quota of junior doctors. The family doctor and his nurses and health visitors are extremely important in providing help for old people, but cannot be integral members of the nuclear team for fairly obvious reasons. Failing this type of membership they must have very close ties with the team, as must home helps, voluntary workers and all the others who provide valuable help.

The team should operate both in the hospital and in the community and have as minimum facilities one or more day hospitals, in-patient hospital accommodation and the usual hospital ancillary services, plus involvement in other types of residential accommodation such as old people's homes and group homes. The team should, if possible, cross the boundaries between hospital and local authority services so that local authority social workers can be as much members of the team as the nurses or doctors. This is not always possible but where it is impossible the team must operate very closely with the local authority personnel.

It is sometimes said that the idea of a therapeutic team is the creation of doctors who wish to collect around them a group of people who will do all the work while they remain firmly in charge. Some teams may operate in this way but it is not the best way. Members of the team should work together as equals and if there is a leader he or she should take on this role because this is the corporate decision of the team. Such a leader should not expect to retain this role permanently since changing circumstances may make it necessary for the leadership to be taken over by someone from a different discipline. Within the team there should not be too much concern with narrow concepts of role. Each member should contribute what he can, which may mean that a nurse or social worker may at times do things that are traditionally looked upon as the preserve of the doctor. At St. Francis Hospital, Haywards Heath, an experiment was carried out in which a nursing officer took over the responsibility for organising the therapeutic milieu of one ward. This experiment clearly showed that a senior nurse could carry out most duties of a doctor as successfully and in some cases more successfully than some doctors. The important thing demonstrated by the experiment was the significant role senior nurses can and should play in creating and maintaining the various therapeutic programmes that are so essential if a ward is to help patients and not destroy them.

It is traditional to consider services as either hospital or community based. This is unsatisfactory since it perpetuates the barriers that exist between the hospital and the community. Having said this it is still necessary, because of present reality, to consider hospital and community services separately while accepting that the line between them is rapidly fading.

Hospital and community services

Figures 1 and 2 illustrate the sort of help that should be available to old people in the hospital and in the community. The two-way arrows in Figure 1 emphasise the fluid nature of this help and make clear that no type of provision must of necessity be until death.

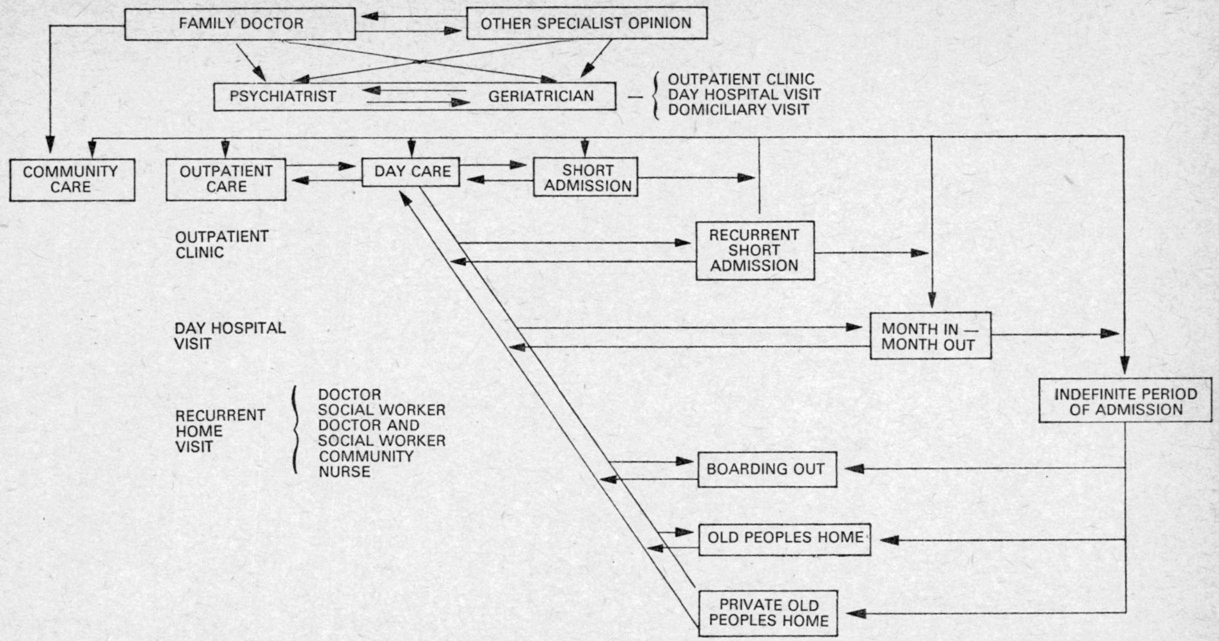

FIG. 1. HELP AVAILABLE FOR PATIENTS AND RELATIVES

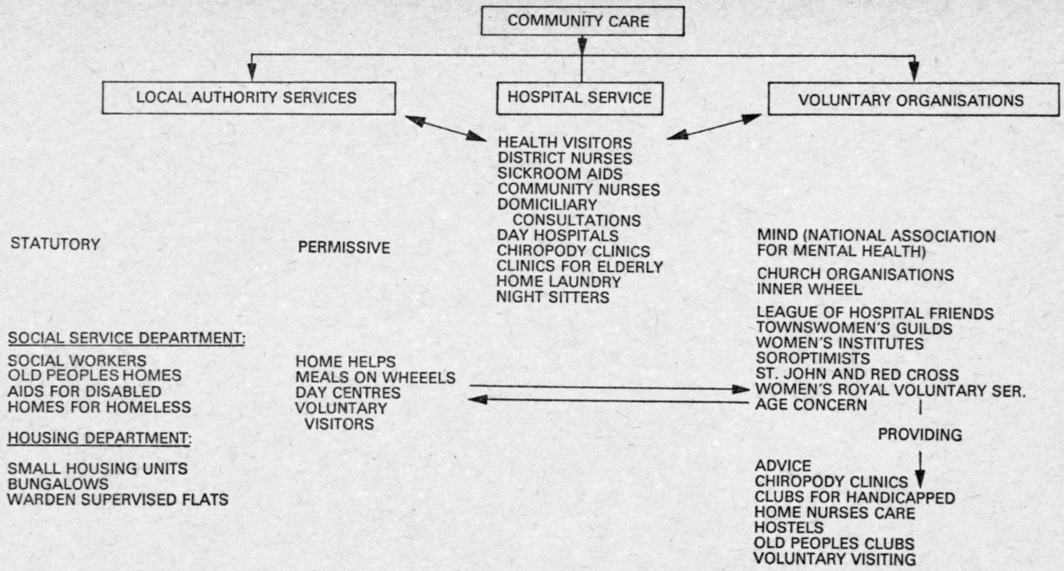

FIG. 2. COMMUNITY SERVICES

The idea of permanent institutional care should not be part of the team's philosophy, although obviously some patients do unfortunately end up in permanent care.

The team is likely to be hospital based and its excursions into the community should be to augment and assist those services that are permanently based in the community. Figure 2 shows what facilities should exist and the authorities that control them. The day hospital should be the centre and mainstay of the hospital team's community commitment and using this as a base team members should visit patients in their own homes, where their expertise can be of considerable help. Another important contribution of the team is the provision of an emergency service.

Emergency service

Patients are often referred for admission because of some crisis. This may be the development of acute symptoms of either organic or psychological origin or because of acute social problems. These crises can of course occur at any time and be difficult to deal with. They are particularly difficult if they occur in the evenings or at weekends, when most community services are no longer available and it is usual for such crises to lead to admission to hospital. Admission may be used as an immediate solution in the belief that things can be quickly sorted out and the old person returned home. This can be a rash, optimistic hope since it is very easy to admit and often remarkably difficult to discharge.

Some patients make their way to Accident and Emergency Departments when they are troubled, or in need of help. Others are taken there by relatives or friends, or sent there by their family doctor. Since Accident and Emergency Departments are not staffed or equipped to deal with psychiatric disorders, the chances are that the mentally ill who arrive at such departments are either rejected or admitted to a psychiatric unit, or hospital.

Emergency facilities for the physically ill or injured are a well established part of the hospital service, yet with a few notable exceptions nothing is provided for the mentally ill. There is a clear need to provide psychiatric facilities within every Accident and Emergency Department, so that the mentally ill who come to these departments can be adequately helped with kindness and understanding. The provision of such a psychiatric presence in an Accident and Emergency Department would go some of the way to providing a Crisis Intervention Service. All that needs to be done is to appoint a group of appropriately qualified and motivated psychiatric nurses to each Accident and Emergency Department and give them a room or two in which they can work. They would need to be backed up, of course, by a psychiatric registrar and consultant psychiatrist on call and have available the normal sort of psychiatric services which will be described in this chapter.

As well as providing this type of emergency service, it is also essential that help can be given in the home twenty-four hours a day, seven days a week. For this to be done an emergency team needs to be established, which is available to go out at any time of the day or night and attempt to deal with the situation without admitting the patient.

Such a facility was developed at Severalls Hospital in Colchester. Volunteers consisting of doctors, nurses, social workers and other hospital staff were recruited and a list compiled. When a crisis situation arose people from the list who were on duty were collected together and went out to the old person's home using either a staff member's car or a local authority ambulance. An ambulance was used if it was thought likely that admission would be necessary. It was usual to send out a doctor with one or two nurses and a social worker, or two nurses, or a nurse and a social worker, or on occasion, one individual. They would go prepared to deal with the situation regardless of its nature so provision was made for them to have available emergency supplies of food, household essentials plus a range of medicines and medical equipment. Arrangements were also made with the local authority for a team member to act as a night sitter if this was necessary.

The provision of this emergency facility resulted in a large number of crisis situations being dealt with without admitting the patients to hospital and yet not exposing them to any danger, distress or discomfort. It was found that the majority required day hospital care once the crisis was over while some, of course, were already attending the day hospital when things went amiss.

Napsbury Hospital in Hertfordshire has now a well-established system for dealing with emergencies in the home, and the staff of any hospital can set up such a service provided they are motivated towards doing so, and are willing to carry out rather careful negotiations with the various organisations that are involved, including the Ambulance Service and the Social Service Department.

The day hospital

It has already been said that the centre of the service should be the day hospital. An effective day hospital can provide all the facilities of a good in-patient unit, except for the beds. This means that patients can be assessed, treated and supported whilst still remaining in their own homes. It may be said that removing an old person from his own home to the day hospital is as damaging and potentially as dangerous as admitting him to hospital. This is never the case. To spend the day in a strange establishment but return to the familiar surroundings of the home in the evenings is rarely disturbing since it is similar in many respects to normal previous experience. Men and many women go out to work, which is similar to attending a day hospital in the sense of being a change of environment. Other reasons for being away from home, including shopping expeditions or trips to coast, country or city, are a common experience to most people, so that the daily going away and returning associated with day patient care is not an unfamiliar ritual.

Day hospitals as distinct from day centres are staffed by doctors and nurses, and provide the normal range of medical and nursing therapies. They also should provide the occupation, entertainment, companionship and meals that a good day centre provides. Ideally, the day hospital should be closely associated with a local authority day centre so there can be a free flow of patients between the two facilities, depending on the varying needs of the individual patient. Much has been written about combined assessment units for old people. These do have a place but the idea that an old person can be assessed as to his needs and then neatly placed in the right niche is a myth. The condition and needs of the individual patient can change from week to week, if not from day to day. An old lady may become depressed and require treatment at the day hospital, including perhaps ECT. Recovering from depression she may still require the support and company of a day centre. At a later date there may be a recurrence of her depressive symptoms requiring a temporary return to the day hospital.

Old people who attend day hospitals usually require transport, which is provided by the Ambulance Service. To make a success of day hospital care it is essential to gain the co-operation and confidence of the Ambulance Service, since without this service day care is impossible. Sometimes the patient may put difficulties in the way of attending the day hospital or may not be ready when the ambulance arrives. The solution to this problem is to arrange for a nurse from the day hospital to be available to go out and deal with these problems, either travelling in the ambulance or in her own car depending on the local circumstances and the geographical relationship between the day hospital, the ambulance depôt and the patient's home. This is an extremely important provision and its lack can lead to failure of day care for many patients, with all the dire results of such a failure.

Group homes and boarding out

It has been rightly stated that the most important single factor involved in keeping a patient permanently in a psychiatric hospital is the absence of a home to which he or she can go. Many patients are admitted to hospital because they have no home, and large numbers remain there permanently because accommodation in the community cannot be found for them. As far as the elderly are concerned, the usual cry is for more old people's homes. This is only a partial answer to the problem; a much better solution is to provided group homes and develop a boarding-out scheme.

Group homes

The setting up of group homes is now a well-established method of providing accommodation in the community for mentally ill individuals who for one reason or another are homeless, or are better away from what home may exist. Group homes are usually set up by voluntary organisations, but there are no satisfactory reasons why official agencies should not do the same. The usual method is to either rent or buy a house and then settle patients in it, who pay rent out of their pension, social security benefit, or wages. This money is then used to pay the rent or mortgage on the house and any left over is saved so that another house can be established. In this way a number of homes can be set up over a reasonably short period.

Patients who go into group homes should firstly want to leave hospital and take up such accommodation and secondly be offered an opportunity, within the hospital, to live in a group situation before going out to the real group home. To do this the hospital needs a house in which patients can try out their ability to live away from the support of the hospital and mix, or otherwise, with the other residents while still within easy reach of help and support by hospital staff. This preparation for moving into a group home could be used for both in-patients and patients in the community who would benefit from a group home life.

The residents of group homes are essentially self-supporting and self-sufficient, but can obtain help and support from the usual community facilities. It is essential that one or more professional workers take on the establishment and support of group homes as a specific project.

It may be argued that group homes may be satisfactory for younger patients, but are not appropriate for the elderly. This is untrue and in fact one of the first group homes established in one town was one for elderly patients, and its success stimulated the establishment of other homes for both younger patients and older people.

Boarding out

A boarding-out scheme is relatively easy to establish. It consists of advertising for accommodation in private homes where the patient will become part of the family. Such a scheme has operated at Gheel in Belgium since the Middle Ages and many boarding-out programmes are now established in the United Kingdom. To be successful, it is important that applicants are quickly visited when they apply so they do not lose interest and are assessed with a specific patient in mind. There should be careful matching of family with patient and the patient should be introduced to the family over a period so they get to know each other before the patient is finally discharged from hospital. After discharge it is often necessary to provide support for both the family and the patient, including day hospital care, and even when little support is necessary a worker from the hospital should visit occasionally to see that things are going satisfactorily. The actual personnel involved in boarding out can be either social workers or nurses, depending on the local situation. Experience of both methods suggests that they are equally successful.

Boarding out can not only be used for long-stay patients but can be employed as a method of dealing with recently referred patients who have lost their place in the community for one reason or another. As would be expected the long-stay patients present many fewer problems than the more recent admissions or those boarded out direct from the community.

The in-patient unit

Thus far, the community provisions have been considered. These services are essential but their development should not distract from the provision of therapeutically-active in-patient services. It has been emphasised that old people can be damaged by admission to hospital. This damage can be minimised and even prevented if the regime within the hospital is a positive therapeutic one.

In-patient wards should have relatively small numbers of patients, never going above 35 per ward, and be situated on the ground floor. Aside from conventional treatment each ward should develop a programme of occupation and activity that fills the day but allows for choice and for periods of rest. Special attention should be given to providing patients with properly-fitting and attractive clothing, preferably their own, ensuring that they wear their dentures and their spectacles and use their hearing aids. Patients should be asked to do things, not told, and always be given the chance to choose when choice is possible.

Perhaps the most important factor in providing an effective therapeutic milieu in a ward is the attitude of the staff. The right attitudes can be engendered by programmes of education, visits to other establishments that have developed effective regimes, by example, and by the establishment of a regime in which everyone can say what he thinks and there is free communication in all directions. All grades of staff from the senior nurse to the porter, and including telephonists and other lay workers, should be encouraged to feel involved in the service. This can be done by listening to what they have to say, acting on it if appropriate and encouraging staff members to think up and work through projects of their own. Regular staff and staff/patient meetings are essential and the person in charge of the unit should make a point of regularly visiting the wards in excess of his normal clinical commitment to talk informally to staff members about their problems, fears and ideas.

At the present time most in-patient units for the elderly mentally ill are sited in psychiatric hospitals. These are not the best places for them to be and it is important that plans are made to establish in-patient units within the general hospital complex. There is an urgent need to do this for a number of reasons. Mental hospitals are becoming geriatric ghettos and while treatment units for younger patients are being established in general hospitals, the old are still being sent to mental hospitals which are becoming demoralised repositories for society's rejects. Most old people have a dread of going into a mental hospital and the mental hospital is usually many miles from the homes of its patients. Geriatric psychiatry needs to have very close links with geriatric medicine and to make this possible it is necessary to have the psychiatric facilities close to the local department of geriatric medicine.

For all these reasons and many more, facilities must be found within the general hospital complex to accommodate all old people in need of hospital type treatment and care. In Brighton it has been possible to do this and the effects have been dramatic. In spite of Brighton having a disproportionate number of old people, the number of elderly patients within the mental hospital facilities and the general hospital unit has been dramatically reduced. At the same time, many more old people have been helped, treated and supported. All this has been made possible by developing day care, establishing a general hospital unit and running the service closely with both the local department of geriatric medicine and the various community services.

Mental hospitals have always been pretty dreadful places, even when modernised and liberalised. The movement towards replacing them by facilities in the community and within the general hospital complex must continue until every mental hospital in the country is closed and bulldozed to the ground. At the present time there is the beginnings of a counter-movement towards maintaining mental hospitals in their glorious isolation. It is important that all workers in the field of mental health resist this movement and ensure that it never gains ground.

Since some patients have to come into hospital, it is important that admission when it occurs is planned and never just happens.

There are three main reasons for admission:

1. the patient may require treatment that is not possible outside hospital;
2. the behaviour of the patient may be such that in-patient care on a short or, less commonly, long-term basis is the only way of dealing with it at the moment; or
3. relatives who are supporting a patient may either require a rest, a holiday or relief when they go into hospital themselves — admission of the patient may be necessary for these reasons in spite of the potential dangers of such an admission.

As far as possible no patient should be admitted without previously being assessed in her own home and every effort made to support her there. When admission does occur it should be made clear to all involved that this is expected to be for only a relatively short period and ideally the actual period should be specified. Before admission it is essential to make every effort to ensure that following admission the patient's niche in the community will not disappear. Explaining to relatives or friends that the admission is only for a short time and doing what can be done to ensure that the room, flat or house will not be occupied by someone else goes a long way to improving the chances of a successful discharge. When admission is resisted it is important that effective help is offered and supplied. Refusing admission but doing nothing else hardly helps the patient and enrages the family doctor, the relatives and whoever else is involved with the patient and believes that admission may be necessary.

This has been a brief outline of the type of hospital facilities that should be provided for the elderly mentally ill. Specific psychiatric disorders can now be considered.

CHAPTER 5

Affective Disorders

TRADITIONALLY, the term affective disorders is used to describe a group of mental illnesses in which there is a primary disturbance of affect which varies between the poles of cheerfulness and sadness. Kraepelin's term 'manic depressive insanity' described this condition. The classical condition is one in which the patient suffers from cycles of illness, in which at one time he is depressed, at another time he is 'normal' and then elated, or manic. This sort of pattern exists but most sufferers from depression, or mania, do not conform. Some people have one isolated attack of depression in a lifetime, while others may have an isolated attack of mania. On the other hand, some people have recurrent attacks of severe depression without ever developing mania and a few have recurrent attacks of mania without ever becoming depressed. Again, various types of depression are described which differ from the depression of manic-depressive psychoses. In this chapter depression in its various forms and guises will be briefly described and illustrated, together with the condition of mania and in its milder form, hypomania. Another condition which is a slightly bizarre mixture of both depression and mania occurring almost simultaneously will also be described because of its occurrence, particularly in elderly people.

Depression in its various forms is more common among the poor and the old than among any other groups. The belief that wealth is no barrier to illness is untrue: wealth does appear to keep depression, at least partly, at bay.

Not only is depression prevalent among the elderly, but unfortunately it is often missed and since severe depression can be perhaps one of the most distressing illnesses anyone can suffer it is of considerable importance that its presence be always discovered so that it can be treated. Treatment is usually successful and even in the minority in which it is not, relief is always possible.

Classification of depression There are a number of classifications of depression but it is usual to talk of three main types:

1. mild mood disorders;
2. reactive and neurotic depressions; and
3. severe depressions.

Mild mood disorders

Old people with mild depressive symptoms are not usually seen by psychiatrists, or even by their family doctor, and there is little published data about them. They tend to feel unhappy because of circumstances, such as financial difficulties, lack of purpose, unsatisfactory retirement, sexual difficulties or loss or relatives and old friends. Bereavement is a well-known cause of mild depression and this is a little better documented.

Grief, because of loss, be it of a spouse, a friend a job or money, is a normal reaction which should not be treated medically, but does require the sympathy and the help that a friend or a near relative can, and usually does, give. The lonely and the isolated do require professional help because they are lonely and isolated, but the help that is provided should be similar to that which would be given by the friend or relative. Sometimes these normal manifestations of grief develop into more serious depressive illnesses. When this happens, specific treatment is called for.

Neurotic and reactive depressions

Some psychiatrists look upon neurotic and reactive as interchangeable terms, while others confine the term neurotic to cases in which depression occurs against a background of a well-established neurotic reaction, such as obsessional or phobic states, and use reactive to describe cases where depression follows or occurs with bereavement, loss, serious social difficulties or some other evident precipitating factor. One disadvantage of using the term reactive is that many patients with severe psychotic depression have features in their history that would suggest that they became depressed due to circumstance. This may discourage the doctor from giving the specific treatment and instead only pay attention to trying to correct the environmental factors. These of course require attention, but not on their own.

There is a division of opinion in psychiatry whether neurotic and reactive, if the latter term is used, types of depression are different in quality or degree from psychotic depression. Some consider that psychotic depression is simply a more serious manifestation of the same condition, while others believe that they are two quite distinct entities. Careful investigations carried out by different workers have shown that both these views are correct which, of course, is impossible. Perhaps this is an academic argument, but it will be discussed again later in the chapter.

Returning to neurotic and reactive depressions, it can be said that, regardless of arguments about the separateness of these two entities, there are many similarities between them. The sufferer usually complains of feeling unhappy, has difficulty in getting off to sleep and may feel worse under certain specific conditions. There may be somatic complaints (which can be more prominent in the patient's history than disturbance of mood), and anxiety obsessional or phobic symptoms.

Severe depression

Endogenous or psychotic depression is typified by subjective feelings of great misery, particularly in the mornings, mental and physical slowing, sleep disturbance, usually manifest in early morning awakening, loss of appetite and weight, constipation, loss of interest and the ability to concentrate, morbid thoughts, delusional beliefs and agitation. There may be other somatic complaints and some patients experience hallucinations.

Severe depression in the elderly may present itself in a variety of ways. Mental and motor retardation may be so marked that the patient is mute and immobile. This can be mistaken for catatonic schizophrenia or, very mistakenly, for severe dementia. When retardation is not so severe, the patient may answer questions, but after such delay that another, or even more questions, may have been asked. This again can give the impression of dementia, since the questions and answers become so muddled that individual answers appear completely irrelevant. More usually the patients answer 'I don't know' to even the simplest question. This can help to differentiate depression from dementia, since sufferers from the latter usually give some kind of answer, however incorrect. Slowing can not only give the impression of dementia, but can be dismissed as being due to normal ageing. Slowing can be a prominent feature of myxoedema and this condition can be mistaken for depression and vice versa. Both conditions can occur in the same patient, when there may be considerable difficulty in making both diagnoses correctly. Tremor, depression and retardation may mimic Parkinsonism and tremor, loss of weight and agitation can look like thyrotoxicosis.

When agitation is a prominent feature of depression, it is again very easy to make the mistake of diagnosing dementia. Patients with dementia sometimes become very agitated and restless and there is a real danger of associating these symptoms too closely with dementia.

An example of this diagnostic problem occurred in a unit with which I was associated. A lady in her late sixties was admitted three times over a period of four years. On each occasion she was very agitated and would run up and down the ward mumbling to herself. Her conversation was difficult to follow and she appeared unable to give a sensible reply to any question. Each time she was admitted a different registrar was involved and each time a diagnosis of agitation and dementia was made. All three registrars were very competent, but inexperienced in the care of elderly patients. Each time when it was suggested that she was suffering from depression, and would benefit from ECT the registrar greeted the opinion with tolerant disbelief. After two or three treatments she always made a dramatic recovery, when it became apparent to the disbelieving registrars that not only was she not demented, but that she was a very intelligent, competent housewife, more able to cope with life than many younger women. The significant features of this lady's case were the short history of abnormal behaviour in each attack and her facial expression, which showed obvious misery.

Hidden depression should always be considered when dealing with the elderly. Somatic complaints may be prominent and include abdominal pain, weakness, headache, palpitations, breathlessness, frequency of micturition and a host of others which are either the symptoms of anxiety or relatively mild somatic complaints unrelated to depression but increased in significance to the patient because of the morbid mood. Many patients deny being depressed, since they may consider depression to be a sign of weakness. An unhappy old lady may even manage a humourless smile and strongly deny that anything is amiss, in spite of tragic evidence that she is not coping. In most cases in which depression is denied, or the patient complains only of what she considers 'respectable' symptoms, such as headache, abdominal pain or constipation, close observation will reveal signs of misery in the eyes, facial expression, stance and gait.

Depression can also present as an acute confusional state (acute brain syndrome). Either severe agitation, which can be mistaken for a confusional state, particularly when the patient is in bed, or a real confusional state, can be the product of depression. Loss of appetite, can lead to severe malnutrition, avitaminosis and dehydration when the elderly person has been forced by poverty to an inadequate diet for years before being attacked by illness.

Chest infections can lead to the production of a toxic confusional state. This can result in admission to hospital, where the infection will be treated, but perhaps the depression missed. Failure to diagnose depression can easily result in the patient being labelled as suffering from dementia, presenting as an acute confusional state and a respiratory infection. Once labelled as demented, the patient can become an emotionally-neglected inmate of a long-stay ward where continued failure to diagnose depression, and exposure to a regime that concentrates on feeding her and keeping her clean while allowing her no say in what happens, will force her into continued demented behaviour, with little chance of recovery from her depression, which will continue to add daily to her misery.

It must be remembered that old people are prone to multiple pathologies, so that an individual may suffer from a serious physical disease, severe depression and early dementia. Treatment of the serious physical disease will not be effective unless the depression is also treated. This, of course, applies equally to the reverse situation. I was asked to see a lady of 74 with congestive heart failure and auricular fibrillation which had failed to respond to normal medical treatment. It had been noticed that she appeared to be depressed, hence the request for a psychiatric opinion. She was found to be very agitated and obviously depressed, with a sleep disturbance typical of severe depression, loss of appetite, loss of interest and difficulty with concentration. There was frank retardation of thought and action and she described a number of depressive delusions, including a belief that she was to be cruelly murdered because in her youth she had said unkind things about her mother. Treatment of the depression was not only successful *per se* but also led to the more effective treatment of her heart failure and fibrillation.

Severe or psychotic depression can itself be divided into different types, such as agitated depression, involutional depression and, in the case of the elderly, senile depression. These categories are of little practical significance, except that agitation may require symptomatic treatment apart from the specific treatment of depression; the actual label should make little difference since in any event the agitation would normally be treated. The division of psychotic depression into different varieties is not usually harmful to the patient except when terms such as senile depression or organic depression are used. These terms can give the impression of dementia, decay and irreversibility, with the result that active treatment may not seriously be considered and the problem of where to accommodate the patient becomes more important than therapy. This is inexcusable, since old people are as entitled as any others to become depressed and are equally entitled to receive the most effective treatment available. Effective treatment produces as good, if not better, results in the elderly as it does in younger patients.

The following case of a lady with a severe depressive reaction illustrates some of the problems caused by this illness.

Mrs. Ellen Walters, aged 84 and widowed for 9 years, lived alone in a terraced house that she had occupied for 47 years. Her two daughters had moved away when they married but this had not particularly worried Mrs. Walters because she had many friends of her own age who lived nearby. Unfortunately, her friends had died one by one and finally she was alone except for a helpful, sympathetic neighbour. She was a healthy, energetic woman, who never consulted her doctor. The first that he heard of anything being amiss was when a community social worker asked him to see her because she was causing her neighbour some anxiety. Over a period of three or four weeks the neighbour had heard Mrs. Walters walking around the house at night and, on one occasion, she had seen her out in the street in the early hours of the morning dressed only in her night attire. She had also noticed that the house was becoming neglected and the old lady was paying less attention to her own appearance and cleanliness. Worried by these changes and odd behaviour at night, she had gone to the local authority social service department, and, as a result, one of their workers had visited. The social worker had found Mrs. Walters sitting in a chair by an unlit fire and not very communicative. The family doctor, not knowing much about the old lady and finding it difficult to obtain any information from her, decided she was probably suffering from what he described as senility, and considered that she needed to be in some kind of institution. He asked a psychiatrist to see her at home, who discovered that she had been well until two or three months prior to his visit and had then started having difficulty in sleeping, with a tendency to wake in the early hours of the morning and either to be unable to go to sleep again or to spend the rest of the night sleeping fitfully, plagued by unhappy thoughts. He found it difficult to obtain a clear account of what had been happening to her, since she often failed to reply to his questions, or said "I don't know". She agreed that she did not feel well, but would not acknowledge that she was unhappy or depressed, saying that there was no reason for her to be miserable. She tended to take some time before she answered a question and generally appeared to be slowed up both in her actions and her thoughts. During the interview she at times became rather agitated, picking at her dress and shaking her head.

Looking around the house he found evidence of recent neglect, with dust, odd scraps of food, an ignored dripping tap, an almost empty larder and a stove that showed little evidence of having been used recently. Some soiled sheets in the corner of the bathroom had evidence of both urine and faeces upon them.

He decided that the most likely diagnosis was that of depression and that it would be best to treat the old lady at home, utilising what community services were available, plus her attendance at the day hospital.

When she attended the day hospital it was possible to carry out a fuller psychiatric and physical assessment. The physical examination revealed evidence of dehydration, constipation and mild upper respiratory infection, and there were clear clinical indications of depression, but no convincing evidence of dementia.

She attended the day hospital on four days a week, being brought and returned by ambulance. The services of a home help were obtained, who cleaned the house on the day the old lady did not attend the hospital. On this day meals-on-wheels were also provided. At the week-ends her neighbour looked in and also ensured that she had a midday meal on both Saturday and Sunday.

She was treated initially with a course of antibiotics because of her upper respiratory infection and an antidepressant. Amitryptiline 25 mg three times a day was chosen because agitation was a moderately prominent part of her illness. This dose made her a little drowsy and she was still severely depressed after having it for two weeks. Because of this relatively slow response and the danger that continued depression would not only be an added misery, but expose her to both the dangers of admission to hospital and possibly a suicide attempt, she was given a course of six electroplexies and the dose regime of amitryptiline was changed to 75 mg at night. The latter not only reduced drowsiness during the day, but also made a night sedative unnecessary. In parallel with this physical treatment of her depression, she was provided with company, occupation, food and an opportunity to discuss her problems with the staff and patients of the day hospital.

She rapidly improved on this regime and within six weeks of starting treatment was back to her normal self and fit to be discharged from the day hospital. However, it was thought that she would become socially isolated and, to combat this, arrangements were made for her to attend a day centre run by the local authority. Here she made many friends and soon became a mainstay of the centre, contributing much and assisting many other old people with their problems.

Mania, hypomania and mixed states

Mania and hypomania are not common conditions in the elderly but do occur, particularly in the atypical forms. The term hypomania describes a relatively minor type of mania and is probably more common than the extreme and flamboyant manifestation of this condition. Roughly speaking, mania is the opposite of depression with the patient showing feelings of elation, increased activity, including an almost unstemmable flow of words, delusions of grandeur and a tendency to become rather annoyed if thwarted in any way. Manic patients often describe intriguing plans to deal with a variety of problems and talk freely of their own excellence. An important symptom, knowledge of which can considerably facilitate management, is distractability. Patients in mania like to have their own way and may become quite aggressive if prevented from doing what they want to do. A head-on disagreement can lead to unpleasantness but, because of their distractability, it is easy to make them deviate from the path they want to follow. A patient may have decided that he wants to dance nude in the snow and, if told that he must not do this, becomes even more intent upon this action. If, instead of repeating that he must not do this it is suggested that something interesting may be on television, it is very likely that he will forget about his plans to perform in the snow and go off to the television room.

Patients with mania often sleep badly and may have a poor appetite in the same way as depressives, although the mechanism is different. Manic patients are far too excited and over-active to spend time eating or sleeping. A characteristic of the talk of manics is the so-called flight of ideas in which their conversation jumps from one subject to another at quite an alarming rate, the jumps being influenced by what is happening, what is being said or the association of words, be it a rhyming association, a klang association or an association from their past experience. Mania can occur as attacks throughout the life of the patient or he may suffer one attack only. The picture may be that of mania alternating with depression, with or without periods of normality in between. The most common manifestation of the manic depressive psychosis is either one or more attacks of depression or one or more attacks of mania, while the patient who has the classical alternation between mania and depression is relatively rare.

As previously stated, mania is not a common condition in the elderly but an atypical version can cause diagnostic difficulties. The following case illustrates this problem.

Mrs. Anna Maria Cantoni was an Italian lady of 65. She had always been rather excitable but had never suffered from any type of psychiatric illness until her husband became ill. He had been drinking heavily for some time and developed an attack of delirium tremens which resulted in his admission to hospital. His wife remained at home with her widowed daughter. The day following her husband's admission to hospital she suddenly became very excited and started speaking at a fast rate. She said that she suddenly felt unbelievably well, but was worried about the Germans who were coming to get her. She said that her husband would get better but while saying this looked sad and wept. Her daughter became alarmed at her behaviour, called in the family doctor who, in turn, obtained a psychiatric opinion. Examination at home was difficult, as the old lady spoke little English, and it was thought advisable to admit her to hospital. Further examination revealed that she was producing symptoms of both hypomania and depression, flavoured with some ideas of persecution. She was almost elated and depressed at the same time and continued to express fears that the Germans were coming to get her. She was orientated for time and place and fully realised the war had been over for a considerable time. A diagnosis of atypical mania was made and she was treated initially with a tranquilliser and an anti-depressant. This regime produced little effect, except to make her unsteady on her feet. A course of electroplexy was decided upon and after four treatments she reverted to her normal self. She was maintained on a regime of tranquilliser and antidepressant and was discharged from hospital. She remained well for six months and then had a recurrence of symptoms which responded quickly to three electroplexies: she has remained well since then.

This is not an uncommon expression of mania in the elderly: there is a mixture of manic, depressive and paranoid symptoms all interwoven so the picture may appear to be that of acute brain syndrome, paraphrenia, depression or, of course, hypomania. More straightforward attacks of mania can occur, particularly in patients who have suffered attacks of mania when they were younger. I have a patient of 90 who gets fairly regular attacks of typical mania and has done so since she was in her thirties. This lady also becomes depressed and usually knows when she is likely to have either one or other of these variations of manic-depressive psychosis. Early morning awakening is the herald of depression and when this occurs she asks for treatment. A desire to keep buying things is her herald of mania; again, she usually approaches me for treatment at this early stage of the attack. Because of these early warnings it is usually possible to abort the attacks so that she no longer suffers from the misery of depression or the social disturbance of mania.

Sometimes the over-energetic treatment of depression may push a patient over into mania, even when there has been no previous history of the latter condition.

Mrs. Elsie Jones lived a healthy and happy life until she suffered a relatively minor stroke at the age of 63. She made a good recovery from her stroke, but became depressed, withdrawn and anxious. She and her husband, who was two years her senior, lived in a second-storey flat which they had occupied since his retirement from the Civil Service at the age of 60. Prior to her stroke she had done all the housework and cooking, and involved herself in a variety of social activities, including old people's welfare. Following the stroke and the onset of depression she did nothing in the house, never went out and spent most of the day wandering aimlessly around the relatively confined space of the flat, fidgeting and pointlessly moving things. Her family doctor treated her with tranquillisers which had little effect and she continued being unhappy and doing nothing for five months. During this period the husband did everything for her and gave up all his social activities which had been as extensive and varied as his wife's. She was referred to the psychiatric service for day hospital care to relieve the husband, and a diagnosis of depression was made. It was thought that a course of antidepressants would produce the desired effect without having to use the day hospital's facilities, and within a month of treatment with amitryptiline she was very much improved, but was still loath to leave her flat. In view of this, it was suggested that she attend a day centre; both she and her husband were in favour of this and she started attending on five days a week. She quickly regained her confidence and was back to her normal self when, following a brief holiday, she started to become hyperactive. She told her husband that she now had such energy that she wanted to catch up with what she had missed while depressed, which appeared to consist of cleaning everything, including washing every washable article. Her husband became a little alarmed when she started getting up at 2 o'clock in the morning and washing all the bed-linen, including the sheets being used on their bed.

A reduction in the dose of antidepressant and the use of haloperidol quickly corrected this swing. Following the withdrawal of all drugs she has remained well, but is a keen attender at the day centre where she functions more as a member of the staff than a client. This is not because she has remained hypomanic but because she has taken back the role in old people's welfare that she gave up when she first became ill.

In the elderly, as in any other age group, it is important to bear in mind the possibility of depression swinging towards mania, either because of the natural history of the condition or the therapy used for depression. The combination of an antidepressant and electroplexy often quickly relieves depression, but unless used with great care, it can result in mania replacing the depression, which is not necessarily an advantage to the patient and certainly not to her relatives and friends.

Treatment

Treatment will be considered in Chapter 11, but a brief mention is necessary in this chapter. Earlier in this chapter it was said that the arguments about psychotic depression being different from or simply more severe than neurotic depression were mainly academic. The arguments do have some significance when treatment is considered. Many people believe that monoamine oxidase inhibitors are the drug treatment of choice for neurotic depression, while the other anti-depressants are more effective in the treatment of psychotic depression.

The medical treatment of depression, particularly psychotic depression, in younger patients is antidepressant or electro-convulsion therapy or a combination of both and this is equally true in the elderly. However, physical treatment is not enough by itself. Various types of social intervention, combined with exposure of the patient to a hopeful, dignity-restoring regime can be of equal, if not greater, value than the antidepressant drug or course of electroplexy.

Psychotherapy, either individual or group, can be effective in the treatment of elderly people who suffer from reactive or neurotic depression, but other methods of establishing self respect are very important in the treatment of old people, regardless of their illness. They are particularly important in mental illness and no physical treatment can be fully effective unless attention is paid to these social therapies. An active, progressively-run day hospital is possibly the easiest and more efficient way of providing this kind of treatment. Many people would claim that this approach is as effective as, if not more effective than, formal psychotherapy. Certainly, sufferers from psychotic depression benefit little from formal psychotherapy but respond well to the social regime of a day hospital, run on hopeful, active lines.

To returning to Mrs. Walters, who suffered from a psychotic depression that responded quickly to treatment: when her illness was first discovered, she was in danger of being looked upon either as simply an old lady who was no longer able to cope in the community, or the victim of dementia. Her family doctor, by failing to obtain information from her neighbour, came to the conclusion that she was possibly demented and considered that the best method of dealing with the problem was to get her admitted to some form of institution. The social worker who visited may have been equally deceived and, as a result, efforts may have been made to gain her admission to a local authority old peoples home, without seeking advice from a psychiatrist. Admission to such a home could have led to her depression still being missed, with a deterioration in her condition which could, in turn, have resulted in her being admitted to some form of long-stay hospital facility, either in a psychiatric or a geriatric department. The longer an old person is treated as if she were demented, the more likely will her behaviour be that of the dement, or what is expected of the dement, so that the true diagnosis becomes more and more difficult to make. Mrs. Walters was not admitted to hospital, but treated in the community, utilising the services of a day hospital. This not only protected her against the dangers of becoming institutionalised, but also ensured that the treatment of her depression was carried out under realistic circumstances, so that the efficacy of treatment could be considered while she was living in the community. Sometimes patients respond quickly to treatment in hospital, but relapse when they return to the situation from which they have been taken. Treatment in the community prevents this, which is not only advantageous to the patient's immediate well-being, but reduces the chances of being rejected by society. If you have been treated in hospital, become worse again as soon as you go out and you happen to be old, there is a strong tendency for all involved to say "This will never work; she will have to be put away somewhere permanently".

Depression in its various forms is a dreadful illness, and possibly causes more prolonged misery than any other disease that attacks mankind. Depression in the elderly can easily be overlooked, or mistaken for something else. It is important always to look for depression when treating an old person, regardless of the apparent pathology.

Little has been said about suicide. Old people who are depressed do commit suicide and, in fact, the elderly are one of the high-risk groups. Quick, active treatment is the best preventive for suicide and this can take place in the community with equal, if not better, effect than in hospital. Sometimes it is necessary to admit an old person to hospital to prevent an attempt at suicide, but this is rare when adequate community and day hospital facilities are provided.

The specific medical treatment of mania when uncomplicated by depression is one of the phenylphiazines such as thioridazine (Melleril), haloperidol (Serenace), or lithium. The use of these preparations, and their possible side effects will be considered in more detail in Chapter 11.

CHAPTER 6

Paranoid Reactions

PARANOID REACTIONS are based on the mechanism of projection. Projection is a universal phenomenon. Primitive man thought of natural forces as conscious entities which were able to have feelings of good or ill towards him. Projection between men is manifest in the belief that others are experiencing the same feelings as oneself and in a tendency to self reference, that is, to assume that outside events are directed towards oneself. When used as a descriptive term for abnormal reactions, paranoid tends to infer some degree of persecution which is delusional and it is with this type of reaction that we are now concerned.

Many old people, particularly when they become forgetful, start accusing others of interfering with their belongings, stealing from them, or in other ways doing things that explain why they mislay or lose objects; this problem will be considered later. First of all, a condition will be considered that is very different from forgetting and blaming others, and is usually referred to as paraphrenia.

Paraphrenia

The following example illustrates some of the features of this condition.

In 1965 Mrs. Mary Jones fractured the neck of her right femur; pinning was not very successful and a prosthesis was inserted. Osteoarthritis of her other hip and both knees made rehabilitation difficult and she was unable to walk again without the aid of two sticks.

Two years later, when she was 67, her doctor discovered she was suffering from hypertension and prescribed hypotensive drugs which fortunately upset her so she refused to take them, thus escaping the dangers of these preparations when used for hypertension in the elderly. A mild degree of congestive heart failure followed which was controlled with diuretics.

About this time her husband, who was two years her senior,

developed haematuria and was discovered to have a carcinoma of the bladder which was inoperable and he died rather miserably. His wife nursed him at home and this became a considerable strain during his last few weeks. Following his death she had a normal period of grief and continued a life similar to that she had lived prior to her husband's illness. She ran the house, did her shopping, visited her daughter who lived nearby and helped an old friend who was severely disabled with lifelong rheumatoid arthritis. In 1970 this old friend died and the daughter moved to a different part of the country because of her husband's job. Mrs. Jones was saddened by these events but continued to cope quite successfully, although she now had few outside contacts or interests and the only time she left the house was to do her shopping.

She started to believe that an old widower in a house across the road was becoming abnormally interested in her. These beliefs developed into ideas that he constantly watched her, using a special device which she named a Main Drain. She considered that he could watch her every movement using this device and could also direct a ray from it, which played on her private parts.

Disturbed by these strange thoughts and ideas she started to sleep badly and became a little agitated and restless during the day, while to prevent him using his machine she stuck papers over the window overlooked by his house and never drew her curtains back. She believed that he used her mirrors in some mysterious way, so she turned them all to face the walls, but none of these precautions helped and one night she became acutely afraid, believing that he was going to do something dreadful to her. She did not have a telephone and did not trust her neighbours so she hurried to the local Police Station and told them of her fears. They were surprisingly helpful, took her back to her home and arranged for her family doctor to visit. He had not seen her since the death of her husband and, surprised and worried by her condition, he suggested that she went into hospital. She was totally opposed to this but grudgingly agreed to see a doctor at the hospital as an out-patient. An urgent out-patient appointment was arranged and she was seen the next day at the local day hospital.

She was able to give a detailed history, and happily described her delusional beliefs about the old man. She did not appear to think it strange that a doctor was dealing with her problems and willingly accepted his help. Aside from these delusional beliefs there was no other evidence of psychosis and clinical assessment revealed no stigmata of organic brain disease. She was mildly agitated with a tendency to fidget, wriggling in her chair and constantly readjusting her dress. A careful physical examination confirmed a moderate degree of hypertension with a blood pressure of 190/110, signs of congestive heart failure and osteoarthritis of both knees and the un-operated-upon hip.

Some routine investigations were carried out, which included a chest x-ray, haemoglobin and full blood count, blood urea, fasting blood sugar and examination of urine. The results of all these investigations were essentially normal, except that blood investigations showed a moderate degree of iron deficiency anaemia, while vitamin B_{12} and folic acid levels were normal.

Following the initial assessment and prior to the routine investigations being carried out, a diagnosis of paraphrenia was made. It was decided to treat her as a day patient and she rather grudgingly accepted this, stipulating that she could only attend on three days a week because she required the other days to do her shopping and housework. Specific treatment was started using fluphenazine decanoate. This preparation is a long-acting phenothiazine given by intramuscular injection at 2-4-weekly intervals. A small test dose of 6.25 mg (0.25 ml) was given the first day she attended and orphenadrine (Disipal) twice daily was also prescribed as a preventive against the extra-pyramidal symptoms fluphenazine sometimes produces. She had no ill effects from the test dose and she was placed on a regime of 25 mg (1 ml) every three weeks. On the days she attended the day hospital she involved herself in all the group activities, including industrial therapy, bingo, old tyme dancing, and cookery. She joined a small group of patients who were receiving group psychotherapy with a nurse and actively participated in the regular staff/patient meetings. Her anaemia was treated with iron, her heart failure with diuretics and she received regular physiotherapy for her locomotor problems.

After attending the day hospital for three weeks her delusional beliefs started to fade and after six weeks she said that nothing was now happening but she still believed that something had been amiss in the past. Her anaemia was corrected, her heart failure controlled and she became much more mobile, no longer requiring two sticks, but still using one more as an emotional prop than a physical necessity. After three months she asked if she could stop attending the day hospital. It was thought that if she stopped attending it would be necessary for her to do something which brought her into contact with people. Arrangements were made for her to visit an old people's club in her locality: she liked what she saw and became a member. She was discharged from the day hospital but arrangements were made for her to attend every three weeks as an out-patient so that she could be reassessed and given an injection of fluphenazine. She quickly became a mainstay of the old people's club she had joined and has remained symptom-free for the past two years.

Mrs. Jones had a condition which has been given many names, including senile paranoid reaction, paranoid state, senile paranoia, involutional paranoia, senile paraphrenia, paranoid schizophrenia, symptomatic schizophrenia and senile schizophreniform psychosis. The more usual terms now in use are either senile paraphrenia or, simply, paraphrenia. I favour the latter term since I feel the adjective senile adds nothing and may carry with it the suggestion that the condition is in some way connected with decay and hence is irreversible. The relationship between paraphrenia, brain damage and schizophrenia is of great academic interest and has been investigated and discussed by many authorities. There is no really convincing evidence that paraphrenia is a manifestation of organic brain disease, although some patients with paraphrenia do have evidence of dementia which progresses. Its relationship with schizophrenia is much more difficult to assess, particularly since schizophrenia itself is not at all clearly understood. A common reasonable view is that schizophrenia, or rather the symptoms of schizophrenia may be the manifestations of a number of different pathological processes ranging from the effects of biochemical abnormalities to psychodynamic causes. In view of this concept it is more correct to talk about the schizophrenias than about schizophrenia. If schizophrenia is not a disease entity but a syndrome of many origins argument for or against including paraphrenia in the schizophrenias is entirely academic. Without doubt the condition exists and as yet we have little if any idea as to its origin, although there are a number of facts about paraphrenia and people who suffer from it that may, in time, fit into a pattern of explanation. As yet the jig-saw has very many missing pieces. Sufferers from paraphrenia are often rigid, obsessional people with rather strict moral codes, who have lived very proper lives. Mrs. Jones had such a personality. The delusions often have obvious sexual significance. Mrs. Jones believed an old man was watching her at all times, including when she undressed or went to the toilet. She also believed that he had a machine which could direct a ray at her vulva and vagina and produced odd sensations in these parts. Another patient believed she was being harassed by a group of boys who had a large plastic sequin-covered elephant that could squirt a white material into her bedroom and onto her bed. This was so real to her that she begged the doctor who was treating her to visit her home where she would be able to show him the stains on her counterpane. Another old lady said that the Duke of Edinburgh flew over the house in a jet every night and sprayed something down onto her bed as he passed. A youthful old man, who had had an inguinal hernia repaired using a wire mesh, claimed that an elderly spinster in the house next door had an electrical machine which emitted a ray of electricity that she directed at this wire mesh, so producing tingling sensations in his penis and testes. All the delusions that can occur in paraphrenia are not so obviously sexual as these but the majority have a sexual flavour. Sometimes the sufferer believes that a neighbour or landlady is doing unpleasant things to harass them so that they will leave. They may believe that noxious substances are being injected through the walls and ceilings, or noises of hammering, shouting, singing and screaming are kept up continuously to drive them out of their house or room. Others may claim that rather sinister things are going on that are not particularly directed at them but cause them considerable inconvenience and anxiety. One lady (see below) believed that the attics in the row of houses in which she had her home were the refuge for all the petty criminals of the town. She said that she heard them walking about every night and this kept her awake. She also said that the police should take advantage of this situation to make a large number of arrests. She did not consider that they, that is the petty criminals, were concerned about her or even knew she existed, and she dismissed as preposterous any suggestion that they may have made the noise to annoy her.

Many old people are suspicious of those around them and often have good reason for being suspicious. They may rightly distrust their relatives, friends and the authorities. Fears of being 'put away', of losing their home to an unscrupulous landlord, a property developer, or a relative, are often a correct assessment of reality. Sometimes it is very difficult to differentiate between the realistic and the pathological. However, the pathological character of the delusion can usually be ascertained either because of its bizarreness, or as a result of carefully assessing all the facts available and obtaining information from as many sources as possible. For example, an elderly street trader claimed the police were always picking on him, which could, of course have been correct, but the pathological quality of his belief was revealed when he said that they had even gone to the length of placing midget policemen in his sacks of potatoes to spy on him. The following example illustrates how mistakes can be made, particularly if care is not taken in trying to obtain as much information as possible from as many sources as possible.

An elderly widow in her late sixties lived in a terraced house that had been her home since her marriage many years before. She began to complain to neighbours and later to the police that she could hear people moving about in her loft. This always happened at night and she was quite convinced that people were up there. No-one paid much attention to her complaints, believing them to be the delusions of an old woman, but since she persisted in her complaints her family doctor finally decided to call in a psychiatrist. She was seen by a psychiatrist, who considered that she was suffering from 'paraphrenia'. He suggested that she should go into hospital, but she was adamant in her refusal and as a consequence she was finally admitted compulsorily under Section 25 of the Mental Health Act 1959. It was later discovered that a group of illegal immigrants were using the inter-connecting lofts of the houses in her street as sleeping accommodation. When this was discovered the old lady was released from hospital, but by then she had suffered the indignity and trauma of compulsory admission and detention.

Insight

It is usually taught that patients who hold delusional beliefs due to schizophrenia, paraphrenia, depression or organic states have no insight and the definition of a delusion confirms this. This is not true since some degree of insight is always present. Mrs. Jones like many others was quite happy to consult a psychiatrist about her troubles and accepted treatment, although a little grugdingly at first. It would quickly be realised how much insight most patients have if more effort was made to treat the victims of psychosis as people with whom a relationship can be developed and not as objects that have to have things done to them to make them fit our odd society.

Forgetfulness and paranoid ideas

Some people always tend to blame others when things go wrong, or they themselves make a mistake. Thus, a wife may blame her husband if the television breaks down, or if she loses a piece of jewellery, or even a can of beans. Elderly people with this type of personality are very likely to accuse other people of stealing from them, or interfering with their property if they become forgetful. Because of forgetfulness, due to early dementia, they may misplace articles or spend money and then forget they have spent it. When this kind of thing happens, they then accuse relatives, friends, neighbours, or their home help, of stealing. Such accusations cause considerable distress to those accused, and seriously interfere with an old person's relationship with others. Family and friends become alienated, home helps refuse to continue working in the house, and professionals in general either shy away, or ask for something to be done about the situation.

Chronic organic brain disease is the commonest cause of this problem. Other organic conditions can also produce paranoid ideas and well-systematised paranoid delusions. Acute and sub-acute confusional states (acute brain syndrome) and certain drug intoxication are well known causes of paranoid delusional states. Monoamineoxidase inhibitors such as phenelzine (Nardil) or isocarboxazid (Marplan), tricyclic antidepressants such as imipramine (Tofranil) and anti-Parkinson drugs such as benzhexol (Artane) are examples of preparations which may produce paranoid delusions as part of a drug induced sub-acute, or acute, confusional state.

Sensory deprivation can be a factor in the production of paranoid symptoms and there is some evidence that vitamin B_{12} deficiency can, on rare occasions, present as paraphrenia.

The following example illustrates how even a small dose of a drug can produce quite florid paranoid delusions.

Mrs. Jacobs was a fairly active old lady of 83, who successfully lived alone but spent her weekends with a very caring daughter. Mrs. Jacobs suffered from arthritis of both hips, but this did not curtail her activity. However, she occasionally took analgesics prescribed by her doctor. She visited her doctor on one occasion because she had run out of analgesics and he noticed that she had a slight tremor of her right hand. He suggested that a drug would help with this condition and prescribed benzhexol (Artane) 2 mg three times a day. Mrs. Jacobs conscientiously took the drug as prescribed. The following weekend she went to stay with her daughter, but when she arrived she first of all accused the daughter of having another man with her and then went on to say that she was being followed by a man who wanted to rob her, and possibly rape her. She spent a very disturbed weekend with her daughter, getting up frequently in the night and claiming that someone was trying to break in, and later saying that she could see a man hiding in the corner ready to pounce upon her.

The daughter, disturbed by her mother's behaviour, called in her family doctor, who was not the same practitioner as her mother's. He considered that Mrs. Jacobs was suffering from paraphrenia and prescribed chlorpromazine (Largactil), which only made her sleepy and confused. Finally, a psychiatrist was called in to see her, with a view to her admission to a psychiatric hospital. He was able to obtain a detailed history and decided that her condition was due to a toxic confusional state produced by benzhexol. All drugs were stopped and the daughter agreed to look after her mother until she was better. Within a week Mrs. Jacobs was back to her normal self and has remained normal ever since. Oddly enough the tremor noticed by her doctor did not recur.

From this it can be seen that old people who develop paranoid symptoms need to be very carefully examined and assessed. This does not mean that they must be taken into hospital since adequate assessment is usually possible if there is a day hospital and it can be done in the patient's own home, if necessary. It is important to differentiate depression from paraphrenia and also to discover if there are any underlying problems such as blindness, deafness, intoxication, infection, or deficiency playing a part in producing the presenting symptoms. Mrs. Jones was a little anaemic but this did not appear to be a factor in producing her paranoid illness. However, it warranted treatment, as did the old lady's congestive heart failure and osteoarthritis. Old people are remarkably prone to developing more than one illness at the same time. The illnesses they develop vary considerably in the degree in which they are related one to the other and it is very easy to see associations when there are none. Regardless of whether there is or is not a relationship between one disease and another, the more existing conditions are diagnosed and treated the better will be the old person, unless the treatment is potentially dangerous or ill-advised.

Some authorities have tended to give paraphrenia a poor prognosis, but this is not correct and the majority of patients with this condition can be treated as successfully as Mrs. Jones. Some are not so lucky and either fail to respond to treatment or end their days in some form of institution, inadequately treated or successfully treated but still kept in hospital because of loss of home or of staff apathy.

Treatment

The treatment of paraphrenia is usually a combination of drug therapy, with social intervention. Drug therapy alone is rarely, if ever, effective and it is essential that efforts be made to counter the isolation which is usually present. This can be done firstly by befriending the patient and then persuading her to come to a day hospital, or a day centre.

The drugs commonly used are thioridazine (Melleril) 50–100 mg two or three times a day, chlorpromazine (Largactil) 25–100 mg two or three times a day, trifluoperazine (Stelazine) 5–15 mg once or twice a day, or haloperidol (Serenace) 0.75–3 mg two or three times a day.

Patients old or young with any type of illness frequently do not take the tablets or medicine as prescribed and old people with paranoid symptoms are notoriously bad tablet takers. The introduction of the long-acting phenothiazine derivatives, fluphenazine enanthate (Moditen Enanthate) and fluphenazine decanoate (Modecate) has done much to solve this problem. These preparations are given by intramuscular injection and one dose can remain effective for two or three weeks or even longer when the decanoate is used. It is advisable to give an anti-Parkinsonism drug such as orphenadrine (Disipal) 50 mg twice a day to patients receiving fluphenazine since they are liable to develop extrapyramidal symptoms. These latter preparations have to be taken daily but patients usually take them once their paranoid symptoms are controlled. Mrs. Jones was treated with a long-acting fluphenazine, receiving 25 mg (1 ml) every three weeks. Since long-acting fluphenazines are liable to produce extrapyramidal symptoms which can be severe, particularly if there is some organic brain disease, it is important that they be used with great care. A very small test dose, say 6.25 mg (0.25 ml) should be given in the first place and side effects carefully looked for. If no significant side effects result from the test dose it is then safe to go on with a more normal dose, say 12.5 mg (0.5 ml) to 25 mg (1 ml).

Another long-acting intramuscular preparation has recently been introduced under the trade name of Depixol (fluenthixol decanoate). This may have some advantages over fluphenazine since it is claimed that it has less of a tendency to produce side effects and may have some antidepressant qualities to counter any associated depression in paraphrenia.

It has been said that the advantage of long-acting preparations is that they can be given by injection and last for a long time so ensuring that the patient has an adequate amount of medication. Sometimes patients will conscientiously take medication by mouth while refusing intramuscular preparations. I once spent an hour and a half trying to persuade an old lady to have a maintenance dose of fluphenazine decanoate. I was unsuccessful but as I was leaving her flat, her friend asked me if I could give the patient some tablets since she was always asking for oral medication. I prescribed a phenothiaxine which she apparently took regularly since there was no recurrence of symptoms.

The treatment of old people who are paranoid as a consequence of a dementing illness is much more difficult. There is no specific treatment and the use of drugs often increases their forgetfulness and those that are likely to produce extrapyramidal symptoms are more likely to do so in the presence of frank organic brain disease. Small doses of thioridazine (Melleril), say 25 mg two or three times a day can sometimes be helpful. It is also useful to persuade the patient to get out of the house and attend a day centre, or day hospital. Perhaps the most important part of treating this condition is to help, support and advise relatives, friends and professionals who are being accused of stealing. This can be a difficult task, but is well worth while since success means that the old person can go on living in her own familiar environment for a longer period than would otherwise be possible.

When paranoid delusions are the product of some other underlying illness or intoxication, the treatment is that of the underlying condition: vitamin B_{12} for pernicious anaemia and the removal of drugs when they are the cause. Perhaps it should be emphasised here that benzhexol (Artane) is not an uncommon cause of toxic confusion in the elderly.

Paranoid states are very distressing conditions to patients, relatives, friends and neighbours. The majority of sufferers can be successfully treated in the community provided there are adequate therapeutic and supportive services available.

CHAPTER 7

Neurotic Reactions

THE AVERAGE PSYCHIATRIST, and even one with a special interest in the old, sees relatively few elderly patients with neurotic symptoms. This is not necessarily due to an absence of neurosis in the elderly, since surveys of patients in general practice suggest that the incidence of neurosis rises steady to the 30–40 age group, and then levels off but does not decline. In general psychiatric practice the incidence rises similarly to the 30–40 age group but then declines. This could be because the psychiatrist and the family doctor have different concepts of neurosis, but a more likely explanation is that family doctors are less likely to refer elderly people with neurosis than they would younger patients.

The treatment of neurosis in general is not particularly satisfactory. The majority of psychiatric services outside the teaching centres arose out of the old county mental hospital system which was basically a custodial service for the psychotic. The introduction of the National Health Service in 1948, and the Mental Health Act of 1959, have, among other effects, resulted in mildly revolutionary changes in the treatment of the mentally ill and the provisions of services to provide that treatment. However, since the origins of these services lay mainly with the psychoses, adequate provision for neurosis, psychopathy and other non-psychotic nervous disease has been rather neglected. Some areas of the country have the services of full-time psychotherapists and some even have the beginnings of a comprehensive service for the psycho-neurotic, but, on the whole, neurosis is treated by general psychiatrists who may have little interest or time to devote to the very large group of patients involved. In extreme cases the psychiatrist may actively dislike neurotics and treat them by telling them to pull themselves together and do a good day's work. Fortunately psychiatrists of this type are rare but a large number, though sympathetic to the victim of neurosis, are able to do little for him. Considering this general background, it is not surprising that relatively few elderly people receive treatment for neurosis. An experienced family doctor has a reasonably good idea what his local psychiatric service can provide, and appreciating the inadequacies of that service in treating neurosis, would obviously be loath to refer elderly patients, tending to reserve what is available for younger and, as he imagines, more treatable subjects. Many psychotherapists would also be loath to take on elderly people, again considering that they should reserve their limited time for the younger person, who they expect to respond more effectively than someone who has had time to become fixed in his ways.

Experience of general practice suggests that the incidence of neurosis is high amongst the elderly, with perhaps the most common symptom complex being somatic manifestations of anxiety. The hypochondriacal old gentleman or old lady is a well-known figure to most family doctors and general physicians. He complains of headaches, palpitations, indigestion, odd abdominal pains, muscle weakness, breathlessness, dry mucous membranes, shakiness, general malaise and a whole host of other symptoms or symptom-complexes that are all the more difficult to unravel since concomitant organic disease is often present. A fairly superficial look at all the elderly patients in a general hospital would reveal a wealth of neurosis, most of which has gone undetected or, if detected, been ignored. Some years ago I saw an old lady who clearly illustrated this phenomenon.

Miss Louisa Elrington was 68 when she was admitted to a medical ward for investigation of persistent severe lower abdominal pain. Prior to admission she had been a regular visitor to her family doctor with a variety of symptoms but a preponderance of complaints about gastrointestinal dysfunction. In despair he had referred her to a physician who had arranged for the usual investigations of gastro-intestinal function to be carried out as an out-patient. He later admitted her to hospital in spite of all investigations being essentially normal. Following admission to hospital she at first improved in that the intensity of the pain diminished and attacks occurred less frequently. Her symptoms did not disappear altogether and when the ward sister left and was replaced by another girl they recurred with increased intensity and frequency. Since she did not respond to anti-spasmodics, alkalis, minor analgesics and a variety of diets, she was referred to a psychiatrist. Her history revealed a number of interesting facts or imagined facts. She was a daughter of a country vicar and had been looked upon as delicate as a child. She frequently missed school because of various indispositions and after finally leaving school stayed at home to look after her mother. She had one elder brother who was an alcoholic and committed suicide when she was 26. At about this time her mother had a 'stroke' from which she made a poor recovery and needed considerable attention. Miss

Elrington developed migraine which necessitated her spending long periods in bed. Her mother finally died and she obtained a job as companion to a middle-aged lady of intemperate habits. This was not successful and she returned home to look after her father who was becoming rather forgetful. His forgetfulness became worse and Miss Elrington's migraine more troublesome, so that a nurse was finally employed to look after the old gentleman. Miss Elrington improved when her father finally died. She took a small flat which she shared with the nurse, who was of approximately her age. They managed quite well with Miss Elrington's small legacy and her friend's income from home nursing. It was not possible to get an overt account of their relationship, Miss Elrington describing them as being 'good chums'.

Four years before Miss Elrington was seen, her friend suddenly departed, apparently without any explanation, and she was left alone in the flat. It was at this time she developed abdominal symptoms interspersed with occipital headaches, attacks of palpitations, tremors and feelings of impending death.

The history suggested that her pains could be of neurotic origin the specific psychopathology being dependent upon the orientation of the psychiatrist. For about a month before she had been seen she had developed symptoms of a reactive depression with feelings of misery, difficulty in getting to sleep, loss of concentration and a tendency to weep silently. Treatment with an antidepressant that also had tranquilising effects was started and a course of twice-weekly superficial psychotherapy began. After a month her depressive symptoms had disappeared and her abdominal symptoms lessened. Plans were being made for her to leave hospital when she died from a coronary thrombosis.

It would appear that this lady had tended to react to stress by developing somatic symptoms. Her death prevented much exploration of the psychopathology and demonstrates one cause of not treating neurosis in the elderly optimistically. If the patient is soon to die, enthusiasm for treatment is likely to wane. This should not be a legitimate reason, since the patient may suffer considerably, become involved in all sorts of unnecessary investigations, take up staff time without benefit to herself, and perhaps least important, cause unnecessary expense to the Health Service.

The possibility of neurosis should always be considered even when the patient is elderly. This must not result, of course, in curable or correctable physical disease being missed, and any possible neurosis that is discovered should not result in the patient being worse off than she would be without its discovery.

I knew an old lady who described pain in the chest in rather flamboyant terms and became a great nuisance to her family, neighbours and family doctor by calling them to help her at all times of the day and night. When it was discovered that she had a long history of anxiety and neurotic depression, she was persuaded to enter a psychiatric hospital, where she died from carcinoma of the oesophagus.

The elderly can suffer from much the same range of neurotic disease as younger people with, perhaps, a differing incidence of specific types. An individual patient can suffer from a variety of different types of neurosis, but it is still easier and clearer to consider the generally accepted specific conditions, provided the possibility of combinations and variations is always to the fore.

Hypochondriasis

We have said that anxiety is more likely to manifest itself as somatic symptoms in the elderly than in any other age group. These anxiety-provoked symptoms can sometimes lead to a diagnosis of hypochondriasis, which can be a dangerous one to make. A patient may develop upper abdominal pain due to a carcinoma of the stomach. This may occur against a background of abnormal anxiety or itself may be a fairly reasonable generator of anxiety. As a result of this pre-existent or secondary anxiety the patient develops other symptoms and may go to the doctor complaining of these, together with the significant symptoms related to the carcinoma of the stomach. When he complains of a tight sensation in the head, attacks of breathlessness, muscular weakness and shaking, dry mouth, frequency of micturation, odd pain in the anus, sweating and attacks in which he thinks he is going to die, the doctor can be excused for lumping his complaints of upper abdominal pain, loss of appetite and loss of weight with all his other symptoms and coming up with a diagnosis of hypochondriasis, possibly associated with an underlying depression. This does not mean that a diagnosis of anxiety manifest as hypochondriasis or depression with hypochondriacal symptoms should never be made until the patient has been extensively investigated for all the organic diseases that the symptoms may possibly suggest. It is, in fact, important to make the correct diagnosis as soon as possible, and this means that an extremely careful and detailed history must be taken, followed by a full and equally meticulous physical examination. The careful history will often pick out the organic disease if one exists. Once it has been decided that the symptoms are of psychogenic origin the next important step is to decide whether there is any underlying depression. Experience suggests that this is very often the case, and effective treatment for the depression, using medication and occasionally electro-convulsive therapy, coupled with appropriate social and psychological intervention, improves the depression and melts away the somatic sensations that trouble both the patient and the doctor.

Anxiety

Patients sometimes complain of the more typical symptoms of anxiety, but this is usually associated with depression, and treatment for the depression will, in turn, remove the anxiety symptoms. Phobic anxiety states do occur in the elderly and are possibly more prevalent than is realised by most family doctors or psychiatrists.

Mrs. Helen Sutherland was a widow of 65, her husband having died four years previously. She described herself as a rather highly-strung pianist but otherwise denied any psychiatric symptoms or any other type of illness until her husband's death. He had died suddenly from a coronary thrombosis and following this, she became afraid to go out of the house on her own, and also became afraid of being in the house alone. She did not consult the family doctor at this time but was helped by a male friend who, knowingly or unknowingly, used the techniques of behaviour therapy, at least as far as her agoraphobia was concerned. He solved her fear of being alone in the house by coming to live with her, and then encouraged her to go out for increasing distances until, finally, she was able to go to the nearby shops.

She never fully recovered, and three months prior to being seen by a psychiatrist, she had again become housebound and depressed. She had difficulty in sleeping, particularly in getting to sleep, and feared that she was going mad. She started to have attacks of panic in the house and called her family doctor. When he saw her she had a considerable tachycardia and he thought that she might be suffering from some cardiac disease. He arranged for her admission under the care of a physician, who considered that her problem was psychological and requested a psychiatric opinion. She was considered to be suffering from a phobic anxiety state with an associated neurotic depression. Treatment with an antidepressant drug and a programme of behaviour therapy produced total relief of symptoms and after three months of treatment she said that she had not felt so well for very many years. She resisted any attempt to explore her relationship with her husband and friend and declined any type of psychotherapy. In her case this did not militate against treatment, since she responded well to other methods.

Patients with phobic anxieties commonly do not consult their doctor until they develop depressive symptoms. In some cases treatment of depression also relieves the phobia, but for many this is not the case and they require specific treatment for the phobic anxiety. Psychotherapy can sometimes be effective, but it is time-consuming and prolonged. Psychotherapists are usually not keen to take on an elderly patient and the patient does not have unlimited time in which to get better. Behaviour therapy is possibly the best answer in the elderly, and the results of this type of treatment are impressive. It is certainly wrong advice to suggest to sufferers from phobic anxiety that they will have to come to terms with their disability and live with it. This is poor advice to any patient, not least one who is elderly.

Obsessional compulsive states

Obsessional symptoms are quite common in the elderly and are often associated with an affective illness. Some patients have had obsessional symptoms all their lives, while others develop them in later life.

The typical obsessional illness consists of a repetitive thought or action with the generation of considerable anxiety if the sufferer tries to resist carrying out the action, or attempts to suppress the thought. There should be insight in the sense that the patient realises that the thoughts or actions are abnormal. Many patients are afraid that their symptoms are the precursors of madness and sometimes the recurrent thoughts are extremely unpleasant and frightening. I once treated an old lady who had a recurrent thought that she would murder a child. She had been a teacher of music for most of her life and had mainly taught children. She was extremely fond of children and found this recurrent thought of killing one obscenely frightening. She also had a recurrent thought that she would commit suicide. These symptoms had started when she was 19 years old, and had continued with varying intensity throughout her life. On four occasions she had become severely depressed, and latterly had had electroplexy for this. Electroplexy produced a rapid improvement in her depression and damped down the obsessional ruminations without removing them. When I first saw her she was 79 and had recently partially recovered from a fractured neck of femur. She was living in a third floor flat, and because there was no lift, was finding it difficult to cope. In addition she had developed arthritic changes in her hands which made piano-playing very difficult. She had become depressed again and her obsessional ruminations were worse than they had ever been. Treatment with an antidepressant, an exchange of flats in the same house, and attendance twice a week at a day hospital, where she received physiotherapy and was involved in social activities, considerably improved her depression and reduced the impact of her ruminations. She started to play the piano again and was soon contributing more to the day hospital than she received from it. Her ruminations continued and she often asked for reassurance that she would never kill a child or herself.

Patients with unpleasant, obsessional ruminations never act out their thoughts, which are usually totally foreign to their overt character. There is, of course, one exception: patients with recurrent thoughts of suicide may possibly commit suicide if they become very depressed.

Most people who suffer from an obsessional neurosis have a so-called obsessional character, with a tendency to be neat and tidy in their behaviour, their thoughts and their morals. There are, of course, exceptions to this, but the majority fall into the category of the very law-abiding followers of the rules who keep tidy establishments and tend to be restricted in their thinking and emotions, resistant to change and unlikely to have original or revolutionary thoughts. Their personality makes psychotherapy difficult, if not impossible, and the only effective treatment at present available to them is an appropriate tranquilliser and antidepressants or electroplexy for the associated depression.

Leucotomy is sometimes advocated in younger patients, but many psychiatrists object to this form of therapy for anyone and particularly for the elderly. It is usually possible to help most patients by other, less dangerous and dramatic, methods.

Hysteria

Perhaps the diagnosis of hysteria should never be made. Few would deny that hysterical symptoms occur, but usually this happens against a background of either another mental illness or a physical disease. A patient with a cerebral tumour may develop symptoms not directly produced by the tumour and having features of so-called hysteria. Treatment of hysteria will not do very much for the cerebral tumour. Hysterical symptoms range from fugues to paralysis. In the elderly the underlying pathology of an hysterical symptom is often depression, the successful treatment of which usually results in the disappearance of the hysterical symptom.

Occasionally, an old person is seen who has spent years in bed yet can get herself to the door, the kitchen or the toilet if necessary. The original reason for taking to her bed often cannot be discovered and it is accepted that little can be done. This is not necessarily true. I have seen patients such as these restored to an almost normal, active life as a result of being exposed to the therapeutic milieu of the day hospital. They have to be taken to the day hospital in the first place on a stretcher, and this may need to be repeated a number of times before they can be mobilised. Whether or not these patients are malingering or suffer from hysteria is a matter for debate. One explanation could be that they took to their beds because of some incident, such as the death of an over-indulgent spouse, or an illness that is no longer active, and have continued this life-style through habit. The rule with hysteria is always to look for the real diagnosis once the symptoms have been recognised as being of psychological origin.

Grief reaction and reactive and neurotic depression

Grief and depression have been dealt with in Chapter 5.

Personality disorders

There is a certain amount of confusion about the use of words such as personality disorder, psychopathy, sociopathy and delinquency, and it is possibly inappropriate to become involved in arguments about these terms and what they mean when considering the elderly. It is generally believed that disorders which produce asocial and anti-social behaviour become less and less frequent with age, and experience of treating elderly psychiatric patients would support this view. This does not mean that there are no difficult old people, but being difficult does not necessarily mean that the label of psychopath or sociopath should be applied. Some old people appear to be difficult because they have succeeded in keeping some form of identity in spite of society's efforts to turn them into quiet, unopinionated, grateful nothings. Patients are sometimes referred simply because the family doctor, the family or the staff of some home consider that they are difficult. What is meant by being difficult is that they express opinions without fear, want to have a say in what happens to them and object to being pushed around. In these cases I believe it is important to make a clear dogmatic statement that they are not ill, and support them in their independence in every way that is possible.

Old people do commit crimes, although not as frequently as the young and middle-aged. Sometimes they have been life-long criminals and it is unlikely that much can be done for them at this stage in their life. Others come into conflict with the law for the first time in old age, and here help is sometimes possible and should always be attempted. Usually this group commits some form of sexual offence.

Sexual problems

Sex drive and sexual ability vary considerably from individual to individual, and this applies equally if the person is elderly. Some men lose their sex drive relatively early in life; others continue to be sexually interested until they die in their nineties. In the same way, sexual performance may fall off early or continue relatively unaffected into late life.

Some elderly people become worried because of the continuation of normal sexual desires into later life, wrongly believing that this should not be the case. Effective reassurance that they are normal can produce considerable relief. If the drive is present but the mechanism is not as effective as it used to be, treatment should always be attempted. Sometimes psychotherapy and counselling of the couple will produce improvement, but failure to achieve the required results using these techniques does not mean that nothing more can be done. There are now a number of mechanical aids on the market which can be extremely effective in appropriate cases. These include devices for producing and/or maintaining erections and others that facilitate orgasm in the female. A number of reputable manufacturers of surgical equipment produce these aids and should be consulted about them.

Some lifelong homosexuals develop special problems when they become old. The reasonably well-adjusted homosexual can become very lonely and depressed in old age and some develop paranoid illnesses, believing that they are being watched by the police, spied on by their landlady and in danger of some dreadful retribution. They often have affective disorders which respond to appropriate treatment, while others develop a frank paraphrenic illness which again will respond to the appropriate treatment. They may come into conflict with the law because of soliciting forced upon them by the disappearance through death of old acquaintances, while others may become interested in children for the first time. In theory it is possible to treat them for their sexual deviation by using the techniques of behaviour therapy, but usually the best approach is to help them by counselling and social intervention to come to terms with their problems and alleviate their loneliness and frustration by providing the opportunity for them to meet people, involve themselves in activities and perhaps meet others with the same problem.

Some men expose themselves for the first time in old age, though possibly a number of these have had this problem all their lives and either were more successful in getting away with it when they were younger or exerted considerable control, which became more difficult with age. It should be remembered that indecent exposure is a harmless sexual deviation and is possibly much more common than is realised. The majority of women have had men expose themselves to them at some stage in their life but have not reported it to the authorities.

At one time it was thought that sexual misdemeanours in the elderly were due to a dementing process. This is certainly untrue, although patients with chronic brain syndrome can expose themselves by accident and may indulge in uninhibited sexual activity. Most do not do so and the majority of old people who commit sexual offences are not sufferers from chronic brain syndrome.

Love affairs

Most young people, and many middle-aged individuals appear to believe that sex and love vanish with retirement. They seem to believe that old people have not only retired from their job, but retired from life. This serious misconception not only means that sexual problems in old age are never mentioned or ignored, but love affairs are viewed as both abnormal and slightly indecent. Many old people develop highly emotional relationships with members of the opposite sex. I have seen a lady of 83, who made three attempts at suicide because of an on and off affair she was having with a man of 60.

It is important that we accept old people as individuals who are likely to have the same kind of problems as anyone else. When they become emotionally involved with someone else, it is important to accept this and provide help and guidance when help and guidance is asked for. Such help must never be offered in either a joking or a condemnatory manner. Strong emotions are not causes for humour or condemnation. Such attitudes should be left to those who have failed to sort out their own inhibitions and anxieties about self.

Addictions

Old people may be addicted to tobacco, alcohol or drugs, although not as commonly as their younger brethren. Treatment is dependent upon the patient's motivation. Good motivation for cure makes a cure likely, while poor motivation makes it almost impossible. The approach and treatment in the elderly is the same as in younger patients and need not be gone into in any detail here. Perhaps the only point that requires to be made is that many old people become dependent upon drugs, having been encouraged to do so by doctors. The injudicious prescribing of sedatives for the elderly is just as bad as the similar practice for younger people. When old people complain of insomnia, it should never be the first thing to reach for the prescription pad and prescribe a sedative. It may be that they are depressed or have unrealistic expectations of how much sleep they require. Some patients, because of boredom and economy go to bed remarkably early and then complain bccause they awake at 2 or 3 o'clock in the morning. A readjustment of their daily routine can be much more effective than any sedative. When sedation is necessary a hot drink and a small quantity of alcohol can be very effective, while preparations such as nitrazepam (Mogadon) or chloral hydrate are relatively safe if used for short periods (see Chapter 12). Barbiturates should never be used, not only because of the danger of habituation, but also because they can produce confusion and excitement in elderly people, as well as dizziness and constipation.

Perhaps the most damaging to the individual of all drugs of addiction is tobacco since it produces cancer, heart failure and other disabling and fatal conditions, but in the elderly the damage, if it is to be done, has been done and it is cruel to take away from an old person one of his last remaining pleasures.

CHAPTER 8

Organic Brain Disease

THERE IS A DANGER with the elderly of equating organic brain disease with mental illness. Some doctors, including a few psychiatrists and geriatricians, tend to view the presence of psychiatric symptoms in old people as heralds, if not evidence, of organic brain disease. One consequence of this attitude is that more concern will be shown towards the problem of how to 'dispose' of the patient than in how to provide treatment, help and support. Many old people are labelled as being demented when, in fact, they are suffering from a treatable, reversible, condition.

A number of conditions can be mistakenly diagnosed as 'dementia', including affective disorders, paraphrenia, and various neurotic disorders. The problems of diagnosis will be considered in more detail in Chapter 10.

Old people do suffer from illnesses association with organic brain changes but this does not mean that they cannot be helped, supported and treated, provided our concepts of treatment are not too narrow and short-sighted. In this chapter the common types of organic brain disease will be briefly described with a major emphasis being placed on what can and cannot be done to help the sufferers. Readers interested in more detailed information about the pathology and symptomatology of the various types of organic brain disease can find this information in standard works on neurology, some of which are mentioned in the bibliography at the end of the book.

Nomenclature

In the past it was customary in the United Kingdom to talk of two main types of organic brain disease — acute or sub-acute confusional states, and dementia. Confusional states were transitory while dementia was irreversible and usually progressive. It is now becoming usual to use the American terms acute brain syndrome and chronic brain syndrome, the first being synonymous with confusional states and the second with dementia. Changes in nomenclature have not necessarily produced changes in attitude, and patients are still left with the diagnosis of acute brain syndrome and despaired of, when labelled chronic brain syndrome. These terms will be used, mainly because they are becoming accepted and hence more readily recognised and perhaps understood. Acute brain syndrome, like acute toxic confusional state, is not really a diagnosis, but only a description of a clinical picture which can have many underlying pathologies. Chronic brain syndrome, like its elderly father, dementia, similarly applies to a clinical picture which can have many origins.

Acute brain syndrome

Early one morning Mrs. Evelyn Barnes was found by a neighbour wandering about in the neighbour's garden wearing only a nightdress and a hat. She did not recognise her neighbour, in spite of their having been friends for many years, but did accompany her into the neighbour's house without much protest. The neighbour slept downstairs and Mrs. Barnes, still wearing her hat, climbed into the neighbour's bed and said "Why don't you tell all those men to leave?". The neighbour, alarmed at what was happening, telephoned her doctor who arrived and found Mrs. Barnes still in bed and complaining about all the men in the room. During his interview with her and his subsequent physical examination her mental condition varied. When he asked her where she thought she was, she became anxious and then in a bemused way recognised her friend, and asked why she was there. Later she became very agitated and said that she would have to get her husband's dinner since he would soon be home and she had not yet tidied up the room.

Physical examination revealed little abnormal, except for mild hypertension, a small right reducible inguinal hernia and a varicose ulcer above the left lateral malleolus. Her temperature was normal, but her respiration rate was slightly raised.

A provisional diagnosis of acute brain syndrome was made with the possibility of underlying early arteriosclerotic dementia. Because she was an elderly lady it was difficult to persuade the house physician at the local hospital to admit her to a medical bed, and since she had 'psychiatric symptoms' she was finally taken in to the local psychiatric hospital. By the time she was admitted a niece had been located who was able to give some information about her aunt. It appeared that she was a lady in her eighties who had been widowed six months previously. Following the death of her husband she had become depressed and tended to neglect her house, her appearance and her diet, but had appeared quite rational to the niece when she visited her.

A more detailed physical examination in hospital revealed some abnormal signs in her chest, and an X-ray confirmed a diagnosis of bronchopneumonia. Treatment with an antibiotic produced a rapid improvement in her condition and within five days she was rational, well-orientated and cheerful. It was considered that she had suffered from acute brain syndrome as a result of pneumonia. Following her recovery she was discharged from hospital to her home and followed up as an out-patient. When she was seen two weeks after discharge she looked depressed, and on careful questioning it became apparent that she had developed a depressive illness following her husband's death and had not yet recovered from it. Treatment with antidepressants produced some improvement but she still remained withdrawn and apathetic. Arrangements were made for her to attend an old people's club which met every afternoon during the week in a church hall. When she had attended for three weeks she ceased to be depressed and became active and houseproud. Six months later she married a widower from the club.

This lady illustrates some of the features and some of the dangers of acute brain syndrome. In her case the onset was sudden: it is not always so and can come on over a period of a few days. There is usually a fluctuating disturbance in the level of consciousness, with periods in which the patient is completely in touch and others in which she is bemused, lost and disorientated. Hallucinations, particularly visual hallucinations and periods of agitation and panic are typical. If a good history is not available, and care is not taken in assessing the clinical state, it is very easy to be misled into believing that the patient is suffering from chronic brain syndrome.

In the case described a detailed history may have produced confusion instead of enlightenment. It may have been thought that she was depressed and had developed a mixed manic-depressive syndrome, so missing the physical pathology. However, it must be realised that attacks of acute confusion can often occur against a background of chronic brain syndrome. Some of these attacks are related to specific cerebro-vascular disturbances, but others do not have this straightforward relationship. Again, it must be emphasised that this association between acute and chronic brain syndrome must not lull us into a *laissez-faire* attitude to a condition that is successfully treatable in the majority of cases.

Chronic brain syndrome

It has already been mentioned that the terms chronic brain syndrome or dementia can be dangerous labels to attach to a patient.

They mean, or should mean, that the patient has chronic, progressive, irreversible, organic brain damage. There are very many causes of brain damage, some of which are progressive and others which are not. Inherited or congenital diseases such as Huntington's chorea and congenital syphilis can cause brain damage in younger patients, and acquired conditions range from deficiency diseases to cerebral tumour. The elderly can suffer from some of these conditions, but the majority of old people with chronic brain syndrome have one or both of the well-known cerebral pathologies of old age, cerebral arteriosclerosis and senile cerebral disease. Before we discuss these two conditions some other less common possibilities will be briefly mentioned.

The pre-senile dementias

These conditions are, by definition, chronic brain syndromes occurring before old age; however, patients with a so-called pre-senile dementia can survive into old age. The best-known pre-senile dementias are Alzheimer's and Pick's diseases.

Alzheimer's disease usually begins with an impairment of memory for recent events and a gradual deterioration in ability to cope with every-day life. The patient may neglect his appearance and become hyperactive in a purposeless manner. Orientation for time and place is affected early in the illness, and often dysphasic symptoms occur at an early stage.

Various emotional disturbances occur, including fleeting attacks of depression or euphoria. Muscle rigidity of an extrapyramidal character occurs and later in the disease the gait may acquire the characteristics of Parkinsonism. The disease can progress slowly or quite rapidly, and it is often difficult to distinguish it from other pre-senile dementias.

In Pick's disease the condition often begins insidiously, with deterioration in behaviour without any frank evidence of memory defect. A very tidy person may become ill-dressed, and a pillar of society take to drink, theft and sexual experimentation. Blunting of the emotions is common, and child-like behaviour with a tendency to play silly games or tell schoolboy jokes is not uncommon.

When differentiating between Alzheimer's and Pick's diseases, the points to look for are the presence of aphasia, agraphia and apraxia which, while occurring in Pick's disease, are more commonly found in Alzheimer's disease. Parietal lobe symptoms tend to dominate the clinical picture in Alzheimer's disease, while frontal lobe symptoms are more common in Pick's.

Jakob-Creutzfeldt's disease is a relatively rare condition manifest in a rapidly progressive degeneration of various parts of the brain, producing intellectual deterioration, pyramidal, extrapyramidal and cerebellar signs. Some clinicians consider that this, and related conditions, could be caused by a virus.

Huntington's chorea is an inherited disease, being transmitted by a single autosomal dominant gene with about half the offspring of an affected individual developing the disease. However, it is not uncommon to come across cases in which there is no previous family history. The onset is usually betwen the ages of 30 and 50 and the characteristic features are a progressing dementia and involuntary movements of a choreiform type. In some patients the involuntary movements occur first, and may be present for a long time before there is any intellectual deterioration, while in others the reverse may be the case.

The cerebral manifestations of tertiary syphilis are now a relative rarity, but the possibility of this condition should never be forgotten, since at least arrest of the process is now possible.

Thiamine deficiency, often caused by alcoholism but having other aetiologies, can produce organic brain changes which again, if not reversible, are arrestable. Wernicke's encephalopathy is one manifestation of this condition.

The first example of Wernicke's encephalopathy that I ever saw was a man of 67, who had suffered from a duodenal ulcer for many years. About eighteen months before he was seen, the symptoms of his ulcer had become much worse and more persistent. Up to then he had paid little attention to advice about diet, but he now decided that he should follow his doctor's instructions. At that time rather dismal diets were advocated and unfortunately the patient discovered that he disliked most of the foods allowed. However, he did like mashed potatoes. For eighteen months he lived on a diet of mashed potatoes and this appeared to be the cause of his deficiency and why he developed Wernicke's encephalopathy.

Chronic brain syndrome in the elderly

The so-called senile dementia or senile psychosis is usually differentiated from arteriosclerotic dementia. The onset is usually gradual, with the memory first being affected; this applies particularly to recent events, the distant memory remaining intact. Because of the memory defect the patient may mislay things and blame others, thus increasing her chances of being rejected. Gaps in memory may be filled by confabulation, the emotions may be blunted, and irritability and restlessness are yet other symptoms that cause annoyance and anxiety to relatives and friends.

As the condition advances, the competence to reason becomes more and more affected with loss of ability even to do familiar tasks. Some patients maintain a good social facade with an appearance of alertness and interest that disguises the reality of their life. All facets of behaviour and cerebral function may be affected, and there is often parallel deterioration in physical appearance and functioning. The patients begin to look increasingly older, are less in touch with the environment and are increasingly dependent on others to do everything for them.

Disorientation for time and place can appear to occur at a relatively early stage in the illness and can be misleading, particularly in patients who are residents of backward institutions, or live very isolated lonely lives in the community. Simple information about day, date and place may not be readily available to them, so that early mild memory-loss can appear worse than it is.

Speech in senile dementia is at first not affected, but in the later stages it may become fragmentary and end up as an unintelligible babble of words.

The pathological changes in this condition include a variable amount of cerebral atrophy with widening of the sulci and enlargement of the ventricles. Microscopically there is a decrease in the number of nerve cells with some shrinkage of the remaining neurones. Senile plaques and neurofibrillary changes may be found.

The clinical picture in the arteriosclerotic type of chronic brain syndrome is rather different. The onset is often following a cerebro-vascular accident, with failing memory, emotional lability and an inclination to wandering about the house at night. Deterioration in the ability to reason, loss of concentration and other features that have been described for the senile type may be present, yet the personality is maintained much longer and there is a tendency for the intensity of symptoms to vary considerably from time to time. Emotional lability, with outbursts of crying or laughter which appear to have little reason behind them, are rather characteristic. Positive neurological signs, such as an upgoing toe, can often be elicited, and in about half the cases there is hypertension. Epileptiform convulsions sometimes occur.

In all types of dementia incontinence, particularly incontinence of urine, may occur and this, perhaps, more than any other single symptom causes the greatest upset to family, friends, staff and, probably most of all, to the patient herself.

The pathological changes in arteriosclerotic dementia are those of arteriosclerosis with softening and haemorrhages in the cortex and sub-cortex, and granular atrophy of these areas.

In between 20 and 30 per cent. of cases of dementia in old

people, the clinical picture and pathological findings are of both the senile and the arteriosclerotic type.

Low pressure hydrocephalus

A condition has recently been described in which considerable enlargement of the cerebral ventricles occurs, associated with dementia but in the absence of raised intracranial pressure. It is suggested that a reversible block to the cerebro-spinal fluid happens for reasons not yet elucidated, and it is hoped that if the cause or causes are discovered, prevention or arrest of the condition will be possible. This would mean that some victims of the dementing process could be effectively helped, if not cured, by medical, as distinct from social, means.

A debate has been going on for many years on the significance of the relationship of the organic changes to the behaviour and function of the patient. The extreme views are that the clinical picture is the direct consequence of the cerebral pathology or that it has psychological origins with the organic chanegs being almost incidental. Perhaps the truth lies somewhere between these two extremes. Cases have been described in which function and behaviour have remained normal, yet post-mortem examination of the brain has revealed fairly serious cortical damage. On the other hand, very demented patients have been found to have brains with little evidence of damage. One view is that demented behaviour, and perhaps the organic changes discovered at post mortem, are manifestations of disuse atrophy. According to this view the active, involved, caring and useful old person does not become demented, while the individual who loses interest, ceases to take any active part in society and is ultimately treated like an object that can do nothing for himself or make decisions about himself becomes progressively more and more demented.

Much more extensive research is required before we can learn which of these two extreme views is nearest the truth. For the present it is better to operate as if the psychological and social explanation for dementia is the correct one, even if future evidence shows this to be untrue, or only very partially true.

Treatment

Over the years a number of drugs have been marketed as specific treatments for dementia. These drugs fall into two main groups: some are supposed to improve the blood supply to the brain, and are said to be particularly helpful in cases of arteriosclerotic dementia, and the other group are described as improving neuron metabolism and can help both the senile and arteriosclerotic types of dementia. There is little evidence that any of these preparations work: they do not appear to prevent dementia from occurring, or progressing, and even the manufacturers do not sell them as a cure. Sometimes they produce ill effects, such as increased agitation, which may be taken as evidence that they are having a beneficial effect, but time quickly dashes this therapeutic hope.

Certain drugs can be downright harmful. The barbiturates are a good example, since they increase confusion, disturb equilibrium and sometimes actually produce agitation. Thus, the patient becomes more muddled, more restless, and more liable to fall and injure herself. To all this may be added hallucinations, often of a frightening nature, and a general feeling of being unwell. The major tranquillisers can also have ill effects, which can be of a similar nature to those of the barbiturates if prescribing is over-enthusiastic.

Restlessness and sleeplessness often occur with dementia and it is important that if possible both these symptoms be corrected. As far as restlessness is concerned, small doses of one of the minor tranquillisers, or thioridazine (Melleril), may be effective. Sometimes a small dose of amitriptyline (Tryptizol) during the day and a slightly larger dose at night can control restlessness and correct sleeplessness. The sort of dose suggested would be between 10 and 20 mg twice daily, with perhaps 20–50 mg at night. However, it is always better to try simple 'normal' remedies first. Thus, a hot drink laced with a little alcohol can work wonders as a night sedative, while occupation and the engendering of interest in something can significantly reduce restlessness during the day.

It is important to remember that restlessness is not necessarily simply the result of dementia; there may be other causes, including constipation, depression with its associated anxiety, some minor painful conditions such as toothache, or more serious organic disease, such as incipient pneumonia, painful arthritis, or a sub-acute abdomen. Acute and sub-acute glaucoma is yet another cause and in fact the list is almost endless, hence the need to examine carefully the victim of restlessness and dementia.

It is of considerable importance that people with dementia be helped and supported in their own homes, preferably until they die naturally. Admission to hospital or to old people's homes is sometimes necessary, but this is usually due to inadequate facilities in the community. The person with dementia rarely does very well in hospital and is in constant danger of becoming a bedridden depersonalised body waiting for death. Methods of preventing this and treatment in its wider sense will be dealt with in more detail in Chapter 11.

CHAPTER 9

Dangerous Symptoms

THE DANGER is always present that an old person will be rejected by someone. This does not mean that families tend to reject their elderly relatives. In fact most families cope remarkably well and it is the relatively small number of disturbed families that give professionals the impression that younger people no longer support their elderly relatives like they used to do in the old days. However, very large numbers of old people live alone, away from relatives, or without relatives anywhere. These are the ones that are particularly liable to rejection by neighbours, landlords and community health service workers. Once rejected by the community it is likely they will be admitted to hospital, or to an old people's home, where again they may suffer rejection, ending finally in some long-stay psychiatric ward miles away from their home and any friends they may still have. I have come across much more intolerance of old people among hospital staff than ever occurs within families. A senior nurse in a general hospital once said to me that she looked upon it as her duty to protect her nurses from 'nutters'. She included in this obnoxious category anyone with a mental illness of any sort, be they ten years of age or one hundred.

Some people have rather difficult personalities and because of this are clearly in danger of rejection once they become in any way dependent upon others. There are not many really difficult people and the majority of the rejected have developed certain symptoms, which will be considered in this chapter. It is important to recognise these symptoms as ones that quickly lead to rejection, so that the symptoms can be dealt with if this is possible and those involved with the patient can be adequately counselled, helped and supported, so that rejection becomes less likely. Common symptoms that can result in rejection, and its associated misery, include restlessnesses, wandering at night, leaving the house and getting lost, accusing others of stealing things when in fact the patient has mislaid them, incontinence, talk of suicide, and violent, or so-called violent behaviour.

Restlessness

Restlessness is a common symptom of depression but many old people become restless for other reasons. Restlessness during the day can cause considerable irritation to those around them and if it occurs at night, anxiety about their welfare is added to this irritation, for fear that they may fall in the night and injure themselves, or get a chill, or in other ways harm themselves. Night-time restlessness can also irritate people living in the same house or, if the old person occupies a flat, those who live below or even above. Restlessness is often taken as evidence of mental decay so other fears are added to the realistic ones and this builds up to a situation in which there are demands for admission to an institution. Sometimes the patient is not in fact restless but simply goes to bed too early and hence wakes in the middle of the night and, quite reasonably, gets up to make herself a cup of tea or perhaps read a book. Moving around in the middle of the night is interpreted as abnormal behaviour and is often described as restlessness. During the day wandering around the house or flat may simply be a manifestation of boredom. To many people old age means sitting in a rocking chair quietly knitting and anything outside this picture may be looked upon as evidence of abnormality.

The way to deal with complaints of restlessness is first to obtain as clear a picture as possible of what is actually happening and then deal with any causative factors, such as depression, boredom, loneliness, unsatisfactory sleep patterns and the anxiety of relatives, friends and neighbours. Counselling people in contact with the old person is of considerable value.

It is important when dealing with complaints of restlessness that the temptation to use sedatives and tranquillisers should be strongly resisted unless there are other positive reasons for using these drugs. A very dangerous situation may arise if restlessness is treated by prescribing barbiturates, as these are likely to increase restlessness which is dangerous because of the associated sedated state of the patient. This is the situation which results in the patient falling down the stairs, setting fire to herself, or all the other things that people fear when old people wander around the house at night. Satisfying, useful activity coupled with going to bed at a normal time, can do much more than any sedative yet invented to combat restlessness in those who are not depressed or have other illnesses which may produce this symptom.

Wandering

The term wandering may be used to describe restlessness and agitation and also the type of mental confusion associated with acute and sub-acute toxic confusional states. Here it is being used to mean walking away from the home with a tendency to get lost. This is commonly given as a reason for requesting the admission of an old person to hospital. The story is usually that there has been some deterioration in her abilities which caused no particular anxiety until she started wandering, getting lost and being brought back by the police. This provokes anxiety, particularly when it occurs at night.

There are a number of possible causes for this type of wandering, including the restlessness associated with depression, a variety of neurotic reactions and, most commonly, organic brain disease. Treatment must include that of any underlying pathology and the symptom itself. Experience shows that patients who develop this symptom, including those with organic brain disease, can often be effectively helped by day-patient care. This applies even when the wandering from home occurs at night. Once they have been established in the day hospital where they can be occupied and given a sense of purpose, the great majority of old people cease to wander from home when they return there. Tranquillisers or sedatives may occasionally be needed, at least in the early stages of treatment, and these can be effective provided they are used with care. The aim should be to achieve tranquillisation without 'dopeyness' or added confusion.

Incontinence

Of all the symptoms an old person may develop, incontinence is possibly the one that is most likely to lead to rejection. Old people can be incontinent of urine, of faeces or both, but urinary incontinence is the most common variety.

Incontinence is not a respectable symptom and often produces feelings of disgust in relatives or others caring for the old person. The sufferer is also upset and can be catastrophically demoralised by finding that she is soiling the bed or her clothes during the day. This self-disgust is increased by the reactions of others towards her and unless something is done, the patient's progress can be rapidly towards bed-bound misery in some long-stay institution.

Urinary incontinence

There are three main groups of causes of urinary incontinence; emotional, lesions of the central nervous system and local causes.

It is possible that psychological and social factors play a greater role in producing incontinence than is usually realised. Patients with depression often become incontinent as a part of the depressive picture. The same applies in schizophrenia and severe neurotic reactions. Less obvious abnormal psychological states may also produce incontinence or make incontinence of other origins worse. For example, an old lady living with her daughter may, because of the emotional interactions between herself and her daughter, take on the role of child, with the daughter taking on that of mother. One result of this reversal of roles is that the old lady may become incontinent in the same way as a child may wet the bed because of an unsatisfactory interaction with her parent. Making old people play the role of children is a very common phenomenon seen in the family, old people's homes and hospitals. The old person may be kept in bed or, if allowed up, be severely restricted in what she can do. Decisions are made for her, she is humoured, patronised, and may even be subjected to the indignity of being hand-fed, washed and ignored as a person who has thoughts, opinions and desires. The extreme of this condition can be seen in some hospital wards where there may be very devoted nursing, but little knowledge of how to deal with old people.

Other situations in institutions may also contribute towards incontinence. High beds which may be difficult to climb out of, cot-sides which make the situation even worse, inaccessible toilets and problems with using bed-pans and bottles can all force the old person to incontinence. Many old people are shy of asking for bed-pans and bottles and find them difficult to use. Some feel they should not trouble over-worked nurses, and others, when they do trouble them, may have to wait too long before the bed-pan or bottle arrives. Some patients have always used a chamber pot at night and when they are admitted to an institution instinctively look for one under the bed if they want to micturate during the night. This may result in their falling out of bed, micturating on the floor or, failing to find the expected receptacle and at a loss what to do, finally emptying their bladder in the bed. One episode such as this can react upon them and the staff involved so that further episodes of incontinence are almost inevitable.

The prevention and treatment of incontinence of emotional or social origin is always possible, provided the situation is carefully examined and reversible factors are corrected. If there is a specific psychiatric illness this should obviously be treated energetically. Patients should not sleep in high beds, and cot-sides are rarely necessary. Time should be spent teaching the patient the geography of the house, old people's home or hospital ward so that she can find the toilet easily if she wants it. If the patient has always been used to a chamber pot she should continue to have one, while a commode that she can use herself is much better than expecting her to ask for and use a bed-pan. Emotional interaction between the old person and the relative or nurse can be dealt with by sensible counselling and, when dependance and over-protection are factors, techniques to rehabilitate the patient should be employed. The latter of course will include all the methods to be described for re-establishing independence and feelings of purpose.

The presence of physical, or apparently physical, causes of incontinence must not exclude a careful search for emotional factors and, whatever the cause, attempts to re-establish the patient's self-respect are always worthwhile. Lesions of the central nervous system that may contribute to incontinence include acute and chronic brain syndrome which in turn can have a variety of origins, and lesions of the spinal cord which range from the result of trauma to neoplasms and degenerative diseases including sub-acute combined degeneration of the cord, multiple sclerosis and tertiary syphilis. Local causes include various types of prolapse and pelvic floor weakness in women and prostatic disease in men. Prostatic obstruction and urethral stricture may produce a dribbling overflow incontinence.

Constipation can be an important correctable factor. It is doubtful if constipation by itself produces urinary incontinence, but when there are other causes such as chronic brain syndrome, emotional disturbance or other local factors, constipation may precipitate incontinence which disappears once the added insult has been removed.

Infections of the urinary tract are often considered to be causes of incontinence. Again, in isolation this is unlikely to be the case, but when other factors are operating an infection can produce incontinence which disappears once the infection has been dealt with. Cystitis produces frequency of micturation and this may be something that the old person is unable to deal with. Cystitis or other infections of the urinary tract such as pyelonephritis warrant treatment in their own right and certainly should be looked for carefully when incontinence is a symptom. Many patients will not volunteer the symptoms of urinary tract infection unless carefully questioned; they may accept pain, discomfort and frequency as a normal consequence of ageing or they may find it embarrassing to talk about symptoms referring to the genito-urinary tract.

Specific treatment of incontinence includes the treatment of urinary tract infections and constipation, and the careful use of parasympathomimetic drugs such as propanthaline bromide (Probanthine) and emepronium bromide (Cetriprin). The usual dose of the former is 15 mg three times a day and 15–30 mg at night, while that of the latter is 200 mg three times a day and 200 mg at night. When either of these preparations is used care must be taken if there is any prostatic disease, gastro-intestinal obstruction or glaucoma.

The tetracyclic antidepressants are sometimes helpful in reducing, or even curing, incontinence. Imipramine (Tofranil), or amitryptiline (Triptozol) are often used. The dose of each is between 10 and 25 mg twice to three times a day and/or 50 mg at night. Often a nightly dose of 50 mg is adequate, since these are relatively long-acting preparations.

Regular toileting is another useful technique, the object being to establish regular, frequent emptyings of the bladder by habit.

None of these methods may be very successful if used alone but combined and associated with other rehabilitative techniques each can effectively deal with incontinence in a large number of patients and even in the others where total prevention is not possible, considerable improvement should be expected.

Faecal incontinence

Faecal incontinence is much rarer than urinary incontinence but its general management is similar to that of urinary incontinence. It is often of emotional origin occurring in depression, schizophrenia and emotional regression. Constipation as a cause should always be considered since this can either result in watery faeces seeping past the obstruction caused by hard faecal masses or watery faeces produced by the injudicious use of laxatives. In either case it can be difficult for old people to prevent the liquid faeces from escaping, particularly when they are being treated with tranquillisers or sedatives.

Incontinence can engender despair and this despair can result in the incontinence getting worse. A positive approach to the symptom which will include a careful history and examination, followed by vigorous treatment of any pathology and the establishment of an effective rehabilitative regime, can help the majority of sufferers. Action is the very early stages will prevent rejection and the demoralisation of the patient.

Suicidal thoughts

Too many old people commit suicide, but this should not lead to the rapid incarceration of every old person who becomes depressed or expresses suicidal thoughts. It is ironic that when someone is driven to despair and cries out for help by saying that she may kill herself, society's response is to push her rapidly into an institution which she may view as a punishment and a rejection. It is certainly wrong ever to dismiss suicide gestures or talk of suicide as attention-seeking behaviour that will never result in a real attempt at self-destruction. It is wrong because the person behaving in this way or making these claims is in need of help and no-one can be sure that she will not try to kill herself.

Some patients will have to be admitted to hospital because of the risk of suicide, but the majority can be helped effectively in the community. The very fact that someone is interested and trying to help can do much to prevent the suicide attempt, while specific treatment for depression and efforts to combat loneliness and the miseries of poverty can remove the underlying causes. It should also be remembered that admission to hospital does not necessarily prevent a patient from committing suicide. Even in the past when patients who were considered to be suicidal, were constantly under observation by two or more nurses, sometimes being sat in a circle, one nurse in the middle and another nurse hovering on the outside, patients succeeded in killing themselves. This method of constant observation had destructive effects on the patients' personality and is now never used, but they still succeed in killing themselves in hospital unless treatment is rapidly given and they are furnished with an active, hopeful regime. Treatment and this type of regime can be offered to the patient without admission to hospital, provided there is an effective day hospital and sensible community support. It has been repeatedly emphasised that admission to hospital can do more damage than good and the presence of suicidal thoughts does not gainsay this. It is more important to assess carefully what is best for the patient than to be too preoccupied with what the Coroner might say.

Violence

Violence and its synonyms are the most misused words in psychiatry. Anyone without experience of mental illness and mental institutions could easily come to believe that violent behaviour was a common symptom of mental illness and a constant danger in any institution caring for the mentally ill. In fact, violence due to mental illness is rare. Unfortunately, some professional workers have fed these public fantasies about mental illness with the result that the association between madness and frightening aggressive behaviour continues to be accepted. Patients in and out of hospital may behave in an aggressive manner but often this is not due to the disease being either normal aggressiveness or normal aggressiveness made worse by overcrowding and the restrictive, bullying regimes still found in many mental hospitals. Most people behave in an aggressive manner at times and this is usually accepted. However, if the person being aggressive has been labelled as suffering from mental illness, this is immediately taken to be evidence of the disease and a sign that murder may be committed at any moment. In the overcrowded wards of backward hospitals, patients are expected to do what they are told and are not allowed to have any say in what happens to them. Such a regime enforced by nurses who are harrassed, overworked and afraid leads them to develop bossy, mildly aggressive attitudes towards the patients with the consequence that when a patient shows a little spirit a situation develops in which violence is liable to occur and even spread to other patients and staff in the ward. When a violent episode occurs in a ward it is important that it is investigated fully and thoroughly because the superficial explanation given by those involved is liable to be inaccurate. It is commonplace to hear staff say that a patient suddenly became aggressive for no reason and struck either another patient or a member of the staff. Closer examination of what happened usually reveals that the patient was provoked to violence because of a build-up of frustration, being brusquely ordered to do something, manhandled because of refusing to go in the direction the nurses wished him to go or a whole variety of other reasonable reasons for becoming a little aggressive. Many people do not like being handled by others, yet in most hospitals it is commonplace to see patients being handled by staff, usually gently but sometimes rather roughly. When two or more nurses are involved it really should surprise no-one when the patient begins to resist and perhaps tries to knock their hands away. Such a reaction will not be looked upon as normal and the patient will be described as violent and others warned that he is potentially dangerous. In many long-stay psychiatric wards it is only the institutional neurosis from which most patients suffer than prevents violence occurring much more frequently than it does. A normal non-institutionalised man would be lucky if he could spend a day in such a ward without being provoked to some form of violent behaviour. If he has considerable self-control the violence he would manifest may only be verbal, but this could result in repercussions that could precipitate him into physical violence without much difficulty.

These few comments about violence and mental illness apply to all age groups and even the elderly can be looked upon as potentially dangerous because of these fantasies, misconceptions and ignorance of how to handle people as distinct from objects. Having a forceful personality, wanting your own way and firmly expressing an opinion can all be dangerous symptoms.

Unrealistic fears of violence and misinterpretations of behaviour that result in violence being imagined or expected occur as frequently outside institutions as it does inside them. An old lady loses her temper with good reason and perhaps knocks a cup off the table. This is interpreted by a relative or, if she is in an old people's home, by a helper, as evidence of disease and medical advice is sought, often with the expectation that the old lady will quickly be taken away to a mental institution. This can occur in the complete absence of any mental illness, but if the patient has a mild memory defect or is becoming depressed, the likelihood of removal being expected is considerably increased. It is not suggested that every old person who loses her temper is in danger of being removed to a mental hospital. The great majority of families are not so quick to reject and, in fact, are liable to accept attacks of bad temper as normal behaviour, even making allowances because of age. It is the family who for one reason or another is in danger of rejecting the old person that is likely to misinterpret her bad temper. Friends, helpers in old people's homes and the staff of general wards can also behave in the same manner for the same range of reasons. The patient may always have been rather difficult and be a member of a rather disturbed family while, if she is dependent upon friends or professionals, clashes of personality and a whole variety of emotional interaction may have placed her at risk of rejection, which then becomes a reality at the first sign, or imagined sign, of violence.

Old people can be aggressive but again this is uncommon and the majority of patients who are described as being violent are simply behaving in a manner that the majority of us would consider normal. There is no specific treatment for violence since violence is not an illness, but a careful examination of the actual violent behaviour backed up with a full assessment of the patient usually reveals the origin of the violence and suggests possible answers. Patients who behave violently because of a paranoid illness require treatment for that illness. If the so-called violence is the result of depression and agitation, treatment of the depression and agitation tends to stop the behaviour that has been labelled violent. Frustration and boredom may play a part in producing the patient's behaviour, and efforts should be made to deal with the frustration and relieve the boredom.

In general it is rare to hear complaints of violence when patients are occupied, given a feeling of purpose and treated like adults, be this in or out of hospital, while the reverse is true when the patient is allowed to do nothing, is treated as a young recalcitrant child and expected to conform to patterns laid down by others.

Whatever may be done for or with the patient it is essential to counsel the relatives or whoever is close to the patient. Sometimes this is fairly easy but in cases where the family is disturbed, or where the staff of an institution are rigid and reject new ideas, counselling can be a hard and prolonged task. This does not mean that it should be abandoned since these are the very situations where the greatest contribution can be made, provided there is sufficient drive to make the effort. The techniques of psychotherapy should not be limited in their application only to young patients with neurosis; they can be as effective with the elderly, their relatives and their nurses.

One group of patients is worthy of special mention – those people who have suffered a cerebrovascular accident that has resulted in their becoming aphasic. Apart from the aphasia, they may be functioning at a normal level but because of this difficulty in communication may be looked upon as severely demented and because of the extreme frustration produced by aphasia they may also be labelled as violent. An aphasic patient trying to tell you something when you are making little effort to understand can become frighteningly excited. If, in fact, they are just able to communicate some thoughts, this state of hyper-excitability takes away from them the few abilities they have remaining so that communication is impossible. This, in turn, increases their irritability and it is not uncommon for them to become aggressive. I was asked to see a man of 65 who was living in a private old people's home. He had been referred to me because the staff at the home considered that he was violent and potentially very dangerous. I was told that he had suffered from a CVA two years previously but had made a reasonable recovery, except that he was now demented. Examination quickly revealed that he was, in fact, aphasic with little convincing evidence of dementia. Simple guidance to the staff of the home resulted in their making efforts to communicate with him which were successful and, as a consequence, his violent behaviour ceased and from being a feared resident he became a great favourite who often helped the staff with their duties.

Patients who are aphasic and given to 'violent behaviour' are the very ones in which it is likely that dementia is absent and speech therapy will be most likely to succeed. If there is some degree of dementia every effort still should be made to improve their ability to communicate since it is surprising how well so-called demented, aphasic patients may cope once something is done about this serious communication difficulty.

This has been a brief look at some dangerous symptoms. There are, of course, other dangerous symptoms, including those of most of the illnesses described in this book. It can be dangerous to have any symptom of depression, be a victim of paraphrenia, develop a neurotic reaction, become forgetful, or accuse someone of taking your property, when in fact you have mislaid it yourself. These problems are considered in other chapters.

CHAPTER 10

Difficulties in Diagnosis

PSYCHIATRIC DISORDERS in the elderly are often misdiagnosed, or overlooked. Depression, in its various guises, is an illness that is more likely to be missed or misdiagnosed, but all the other disorders can also be either dismissed as the normal consequence of ageing, or their symptoms put down to 'senility'. Dangerous symptoms were described in the previous chapter. The following account illustrates the dangers of having symptoms of depression.

Mrs. Ellen Morris was referred to the psychogeriatric service by a general psychiatrist as a case of progressive dementia requiring prolonged institutional care. She was 78 years old and had first been seen by the referring psychiatrist six months previously. At that time her husband, who was 80 years old, said his wife had been deteriorating for some months, and for this period had been unable to do any work in the house or care for herself, so he had to do everything and she had become progressively unkempt. Her husband said that she often appeared not to know where she was and he could make little sense out of her conversation. The psychiatrist described her as apathetic, untidily dressed, and not particularly clean. She failed to answer any questions except about her name and age and he considered that she was suffering from dementia, possibly of the senile variety. He suggested that the family could be supported for the time being with the usual community services, but considered that there would soon come a time when the old lady would require permanent institutional care. No specific treatment regime was suggested. Six months later the patient's general practitioner telephoned the psychiatrist to say that the husband was no longer able to cope. As a result of this telephone conversation, the old lady was admitted to hospital and the husband told this would be a permanent admission.

She was taken over by the psychogeriatric service and it was discovered that six years previously she had been diagnosed as suffering from depression, and following a short course of antidepressants, had made a dramatic recovery. Following this, she had been well until approximately nine or ten months before coming into hospital. She had gradually lost interest, had difficulty with sleeping, and lost her appetite. At first she kept telling her husband that she was no good and should be put away, but latterly she had become more withdrawn, tending to sit in a chair all day doing nothing except stare sadly into space. Sometimes she had been incontinent of urine.

On examination she was found to be an unhappy-looking old lady, who had obviously neglected herself, and was very thin, dehydrated and had long uncut finger and toenails. She tended to reply to questions by saying 'I don't know' but could occasionally be persuaded to answer, and on these occasions the answer was correct.

She was considered to be suffering from a severe endogenous depression and, following treatment with antidepressants, made a fairly rapid recovery. Examination after recovery revealed no evidence of dementia, and in fact when she returned home she demonstrated that she was still a competent housewife.

There are a number of reasons why the elderly are in greater danger than younger people of being misdiagnosed, or having their symptoms ignored.

Misconceptions of normality

It is not uncommon for the symptoms and signs of depression to be mistaken for the wrongly-believed normal features of ageing. Old people are expected to be slowed up in their thoughts and actions, experience difficulties with sleeping, have a reduced appetite, lose interest in life, have difficulty with concentration and neglect themselves and their accommodation. These changes in behaviour, all manifestations of depression, can in part be due to normal ageing, or to a dementing process. A careful history and assessment of each symptom usually reveals the correct diagnosis. For example, a meticulous old lady who fairly rapidly begins to neglect herself is more likely to be suffering from depression than anything else. Evidence of early dementia or other physical disease does not mean the patient is not depressed. Depression can occur alone, but also in association with other illnesses. In these cases the depression warrants treatment in its own right, since it is unlikely to improve simply by treating the associated physical disease.

The symptoms of anxiety can be dismissed as either a normal consequence of ageing, or as an early sign of a dementing illness. People with dementia often become anxious, agitated and restless and this cluster of symptoms, which of course can occur with anxiety, may be taken to mean something which they are not, with the consequence that once again 'disposal', with all its unpleasant meanings becomes more important than treatment and support.

Even people suffering from paraphrenia can either be ignored or dealt with as if they were suffering from organic brain disease. In these cases, treating them as if there was nothing amiss is not necessarily such a bad thing, but viewing them as having dementia can only lead to disaster for the patient.

Depression, not dementia

Depression in the elderly can present with a picture very like that of a dementing process. Patients who are very retarded because of depression may either fail to answer questions, or simply say 'I don't know'. This can lead the doctor to believe that they are dementing. Sometimes the patient will complain of failing memory and doing silly things. For example, I have seen an old lady who said that she was losing her memory and as a consequence often did foolish things in her kitchen, such as mistaking salt for sugar, and starting to fry some syringes she had for injections, in mistake for fish fingers. In fact this forgetfulness and muddled behaviour was due to agitation and lack of concentration not to any disturbance of memory as such.

The following case illustrates some of the problems in differentiating between depression and dementia.

Mrs. Dora Brown, a lady of 66, was admitted to the psychiatric unit at the request of a local physician. Five months prior to this she had been admitted under the care of a gynaecologist for a pelvic floor repair. At that time she was mentally well, but after the operation she became what was described as confused and very forgetful. Because of the development of these symptoms she was transferred to a medical ward under the care of a physician. Here she was described as confused, disorientated and aggressive. A diagnosis of dementia was made. Thyroid dysfunction was considered and excluded.

An electroencephalogram showed some changes in the right hemisphere which were considered probably to be arteriosclerotic in origin. Other investigations, including skull x-ray and tests for syphilis, carried out at that time were negative. A consultant neurologist saw her and considered that she was probably suffering from arteriosclerotic dementia: a consultant psychiatrist agreeing with this diagnosis recommended her admission to the psychiatric unit. On admission she presented a picture of great misery. There was frank psychomotor retardation and she was unable or unwilling to give much account of herself. She tended to wander aimlessly about the ward and was incontinent of both urine and faeces.

The day following admission she was able to give some history. She said that she had felt depressed at times over a period of eight years, but recently had become much more depressed and wished that she could die. She was considered to be suffering from a severe depression and was treated with a course of electroconvulsive therapy and antidepressants. She improved rapidly and dramatically, quickly becoming a happy, well-orientated woman who was keen to help other patients on the ward.

She spent a successful week-end at home with her husband, following which she was discharged, but arrangements were made for her to attend the day hospital. Day hospital attendance was quickly reduced from five to two days per week, and she is now followed up as an out-patient.

Respectable physical diseases

Many old people are loath to complain of 'nervous problems', since they look upon these problems as evidence of lack of moral fibre. Not only may they not mention their feelings of misery, anxiety, etc., but they may actually deny having any symptom that could vaguely be looked upon as nervous in origin. However, they may complain of organic symptoms that they accept as respectable. Both depression and anxiety are symptoms that can easily be related to organic disease. Thus the patient may complain of constipation and abdominal pain, headaches and a whole variety of sensations which are the result of anxiety. Dry mouths and throats that become sore, an increased pulse rate, which may be described as palpitations, tight sensations in the chest, sinking feelings in the abdomen, muscular weakness and shakiness, and a general feeling of being unwell, are typical symptoms of anxiety. The patient may complain of any of these symptoms, or any combination of symptoms, so leading the unsuspecting doctor towards a diagnosis of a physical illness. Depressed patients may also become more aware of some innocuous pain that would not bother them if they were not depressed. The next case illustrates this phenomenon.

Miss Elizabeth May lived with her single sister, and was admitted after having taken an overdose of sodium amytal. Following recovery from the overdose she said that she had taken the capsules because of intolerable pain in her neck; this pain had prevented her from sleeping for years, and was now more than she could stand.

She had had pain in her neck off and on for a period of 11 years but this had not worried her until a few months prior to her suicide attempt. She consulted her family doctor who prescribed analgesics: these had no effect and she was referred to the hospital physical medicine department where manipulations were carried out. She later saw a physician who ordered a whole range of investigations, including carotid angiography. No cause for her pain was discovered and she was referred to a psychiatrist who considered her to be suffering from mild anxiety symptoms, and prescribed a minor tranquilliser.

When she recovered from her suicide attempt a detailed history was taken, and this revealed considerable evidence of a depressive illness. She was treated with electroconvulsive therapy and antidepressants, rapidly improved and became symptom-free, and said she had never felt so well for years. She now lives a normal, active life.

It has been inferred here that old people may use the physical symptoms of emotional disorders as a method of seeking help from a doctor. Of course they may not realise that these symptoms are due to mental illness, and are extremely worried and concerned about the possibility of a serious physical disease. When the doctor goes along with them in this misconception, not only is the psychiatric disorder missed, and hence not treated, but the patient becomes even more convinced that there is something seriously amiss and if a time comes when it is realised that the illness is psychiatric, it becomes remarkably difficult to convince the patient that this is the case. If you have been investigated by one or more doctors, and the investigations have included such procedures as chest x-rays, electrocardiagrams, and barium meals, it is understandable that you will be a little loath to accept the diagnosis of anxiety, or depression, since you will argue that no doctor would carry out these investigations unless he believed there was a serious organic disease present, and it is well known that serious diseases are missed even when sophisticated methods of investigation are used. It is of considerable importance that a psychiatric disorder be diagnosed as early as possible, provided of course that the person is suffering from a psychiatric illness and the diagnosis made is the correct one.

Psychiatric disorders complicating physical disease

Some old people can suffer from many illnesses at the same time. It is not uncommon for psychiatric disorders to occur with serious, and not so serious, physical disease. In these cases, the better-understood organic illness will dominate the picture for the doctor, if not the patient. Failure to recognise and treat the associated mental illness in these cases is not only likely to result in unnecessary suffering, but is also likely that there will be a poor response to treatment of the organic condition.

Some illnesses such as myxoedema, thyrotoxicosis, Parkinsonism, potassium deficiency and severe anaemia can mimic depression, and when physical illness and depression occur together the correct diagnosis can be difficult. Anxiety by itself, manifest as a phobic state or produced by an obsessional compulsive neurosis, can very easily be overlooked when a serious physical illness is present. Perhaps the easiest trap to fall into is to ignore anxiety in the presence of heart disease. Another common mistake is to accept that the housebound arthritic is housebound because of arthritis, when in fact she has a phobic state and is afraid to leave the house.

Remembering the possibility of psychiatric disorder, even when the patient has some other disease, usually means that this disorder, if present, is discovered and treated in its own right.

The mixed manic-depressive state

It has been mentioned in Chapter 5 that mania is uncommon in the elderly, but when it does occur the picture is usually one in which the symptoms of mania are mixed with those of depression, sometimes made even more complicated by paranoid delusions. The patient may be elated, overtalkative, over-active and express grandiose ideas, yet at times will become depressed, tearful and morbid. When there is evidence of paranoid delusions as well as this odd mixture of elation and depression it is not uncommon for the unhelpful diagnosis of senile psychosis to be made, with an inference that the underlying pathology is that of organic brain disease. The next case illustrates some of these features.

Miss June Williams, a single lady of 84, lived in a first floor flat which she had occupied for some years. Up to the age of 83 she had cared for herself and the flat without assistance from anyone, but then fell, fracturing her right femur. Operative treatment for this was successful, and she returned to her flat, continuing to care for herself without any outside assistance. A nephew and niece visited her at week-ends and always found her well cared for and happy.

Suddenly, over a period of two or three days she became disturbed for no apparent reason. She started to make a lot of noise, shouting and crying both during the day and at night. She moved all the furniture in one room into a corner, rolled up the carpet, and then rushed out into the street shouting for the fire brigade and police. When she was visited in her home, she had gone to bed wearing all her clothes. She spoke rapidly, jumping from one subject to another, and often interspersing her conversation with a few verses of a popular song of her youth. She said that she felt marvellous, but wished for company so that she could have a party. In the midst of this flow of talk she would suddenly become quite agitated and tearful saying that something dreadful was going to happen to her and that already the roof was leaking and water was pouring into her front room. This apparently was the reason why she had moved all the furniture into one corner and called for the police and fire brigade.

It was impossible to get any type of history from her, nor would she answer the usual questions designed to ascertain orientation and memory.

She was considered to be suffering from a mixed manic depressive state, admitted to hospital and treated with electroconvulsive therapy. She made a rapid recovery, returning to her flat, where she has continued to care for herself in a competent manner.

Lack of interest

Relatively few doctors, particularly in the hospital service, have an interest in old people. Geriatricians are an obvious exception, but psychiatrists are not. Lack of interest in the elderly leads to a tendency to look upon any manifestation of mental illness occurring in people who are past the magic age of 65 as evidence of a dementing process. This means that the patient will be looked upon more as a problem of so-called disposal than one of treatment. The case of Mrs. Ellen Morris illustrates this approach. The psychiatrist involved was competent and conscientious in his normal psychiatric practice, yet quickly dismissed an old person, who was obviously depressed, as being demented and requiring permanent institutional care.

There is little doubt that psychiatric disorders in the elderly, particularly depression, are often overlooked and remain untreated. Old people with mental disorders respond to treatment and recover in the same way as younger people. Missing the diagnosis of these disorders means that old people will suffer misery, often for a very prolonged period which may extend until death. Not only is there misery for the patient, but because of the effects of the illness on behaviour it is likely that these individuals will spend prolonged periods in institutions, which in turn has further damaging effects upon them. Their relatives and friends will be distressed and in turn may themselves become victims of mental illness.

Treatment of mental illness in the elderly is in the main no different from its treatment in younger people, except perhaps in detail. There is one important difference, which relates to drug therapy. Old people are much more likely to develop side effects than younger individuals, and it is important that this should always be remembered when prescribing. Treatment will be considered in more detail in the next chapter.

CHAPTER 11

Treatment

THE BROADER CONCEPTS of treatment have been discussed in Chapter 4. In the present chapter specific treatments will be considered. It must be emphasised that most specific treatments are never enough in themselves and must be provided against a background of help, support, understanding, and above all else a respect for the individual as a person.

Figure 3 illustrates the kinds of specific treatment that should be available for the various psychiatric illnesses that affect the elderly.

Psychotherapy

Psychotherapy can mean many things, from a formal Freudian-type analysis to a few brief interviews with a psychiatrist. It can also be carried out on an individual basis or in a group. Many psychiatrists would not consider that the elderly are good subjects for psychotherapy, although some have claimed impressive results using various techniques, including those of the analyst. The effectiveness of psychotherapy is difficult to assess, and in the elderly particularly it may be that any good results have occurred simply because someone has spent time regularly talking to the patient and would have been as good if they had talked about football or the Boer War. Experience suggests that elderly patients with neurotic reactions are helped by both individual and group psychotherapy, provided this is relatively simple. In view of the numbers involved and the relative scarcity of staff, group techniques are often the best and this is particularly so if the therapeutic regime also involves regular group meetings between staff and patients in which broader ideas of treatment and organisation are considered. Regular patient/staff meetings introduce the patient to the group milieu and prepare him for the therapeutic group where he is then able to participate more freely and more quickly than is the case when his experience is limited to therapeutic groups only. Group therapy for the elderly can also be useful for patients with depression and chronic brain syndrome (dementia).

Occupational therapy

Occupational therapy no longer means just making baskets and rugs; it now includes so-called industrial therapy, social activities, household management and entertainment. The occupational therapist can play a vital part in the therapeutic team, providing occupation, entertainment and other activities that restore the patient's self-respect and feelings of usefulness. Traditional occupational therapy can be and is very useful, but it is never enough by itself. Very many old people feel that they are no longer useful members of society and may look upon themselves as old wrecks waiting dismally for death. Industrial-type therapy, in which tasks are carried out of varying complexity depending upon the ability of the patient, producing a useful article and financial remuneration, can do much to restore the individual's self-respect.

Guidance in household management, which should include shopping, cooking, washing and other housewifely tasks many sound like teaching grandmothers to suck eggs, but in fact many patients, particularly those with chronic brain syndrome need this type of rehabilitation and benefit from it to the extent of being able to return to a normal independent existence in the community. When there are physical disabilities new techniques may need to be learned, including the use of special equipment which can minimise disability.

Whatever activity is provided, greater benefit usually accrues to the patient if it is carried out in a group, since this improves the patient's ability to deal with others and relate to and communicate with them.

Entertainment can be anything from listening to records to organising and participating in a social evening and can be as therapeutic as any other type of occupational therapy. The old not only require treatments that will improve function but also activities that bring them in close contact with others and pleasantly occupy their day. One of the most destructive things that can be done to an old person is to take away any opportunity for activity and the sorry sight of old people sitting in chairs gazing into space apathetically waiting for the next meal is something that should never be seen in any establishment for the elderly, be it hospital, old people's home or the patient's own home.

Behaviour therapy

Behaviour therapy is based on the original work of Pavlov, Watson and Skinner. In simple terms it depends upon conditioning and

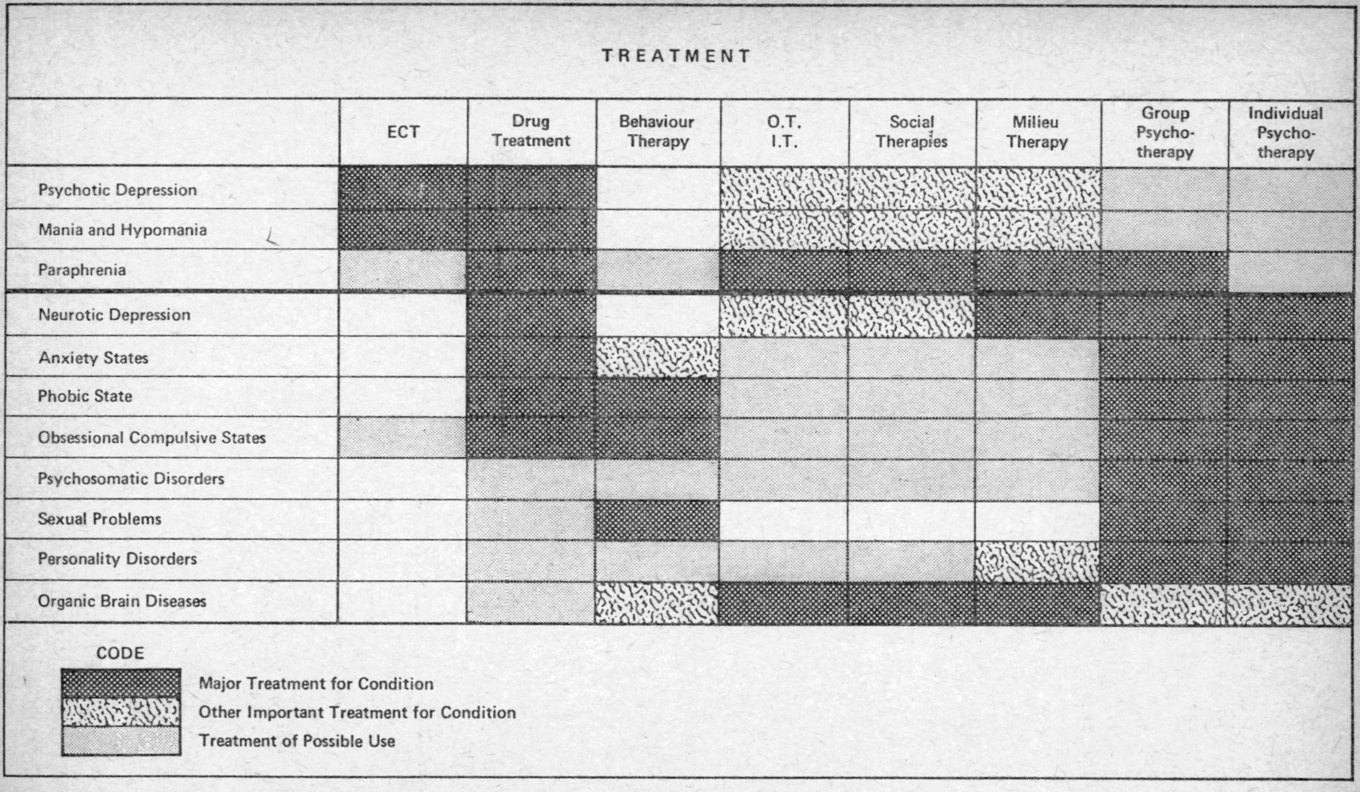

FIG. 3. This figure shows the type of treatment that should be easily available for old people with mental illness. It should be emphasised that no treatment is effective in the absence of other factors mentioned in the text.

de-conditioning. Practitioners who use behaviour therapy sometimes make rather extravagant claims, but there is accumulating evidence to show that it does have a place among the psychiatric treatments. It can be effective in treating phobic states and very many patients who were housebound are now able to live a normal life because this technique has been used to help them. This is not the place to go into considerable detail, particularly since the number of elderly patients who can definitely be helped by these methods is relatively small. However, there are exciting possibilities that variations on behaviourist techniques can be used to improve patients who suffer from chronic brain syndrome or have been damaged by prolonged institutionalisation. I have seen elderly institutionalised patients who sat around dumb and immobile start to become actively involved in ward activities and social functions with a return of the use of speech, following the use of relatively simple behaviourist techniques that were taught to the nurses by a psychologist interested in these methods. This was done by offering patients a reward such as a sweet or a cigarette when they spoke and witholding the reward until they did speak. Once they had started speaking again other techniques of rehabilitation were possible so the patients could be returned to a level at which leaving the hospital for a semi-independent life in the community was possible.

Electroplexy and other physical treatments

Electroplexy (ECT) is a very effective method of treating depression and old age is no contraindication to its use. A severely depressed patient may be in such misery that quick relief is called for. Most antidepressants take anything from 10 to 21 days to take effect, while electroplexy can result in some improvement after one or two treatments, although it is usual for noticeable effects to be delayed until the third or fourth treatment. It is common practice to give six treatments but there are no hard and fast rules about this, some patients requiring only four, while others may require anything up to 10 or 12.

Some old people appear to have a high fit threshold and in these it may be difficult to induce a convulsion. It is important that a convulsion is induced since sub-fit doses of electrical stimulation often produce post-treatment confusion which not only is distressing to the patient but may lead the doctor to stop further treatment or, even worse, consider the patient to be suffering from dementia which is not treatable. Even when a normal fit occurs under treatment some patients do become confused afterwards. Unilateral ECT does reduce this risk.

In the elderly, ECT should be used either because the depression is severe, requires rapid treatment or the patient has failed to respond to antidepressants and other treatments. ECT can be lifesaving since the patients may be so depressed that they are refusing to eat or drink and spend the day almost immobile. Under these conditions they are in danger of suffering the effects of dehydration and malnutrition, coupled with bronchopneumonia because of their immobility.

Other physical treatments used in psychiatry include various types of leucotomy. Many would consider there was no place for leucotomy, and its variations, in the treatment of any patient, and I strongly subscribe to this view. Even supporters of leucotomy rarely advocate its use in the elderly, except perhaps for the old person with severe depression, who has failed to respond to any other treatment and continues to live in a state of considerable misery.

The problem with psycho-surgery is that it is irreversible and usually ineffective. Not only is it ineffective but it can produce ill effects in its own right. Since this is a book about the treatment of the elderly, it is not really appropriate to include a long discussion on a form of treatment that is rarely if ever used for this age group.

Drug therapy

Old people tend to suffer from many diseases and because of this they may be exposed to a whole variety of differing drug therapies. They may be receiving digoxin and a diuretic for a cardiac pathology, analgesics for arthritis, something for diabetes, yet other drugs for depression, night sedatives for sleep disturbance, laxatives for constipation, an antibiotic for some infection and drops and ointments for afflictions of the eye and skin. I would hope that not many patients have this plethora of medication but many are seen who would make good runners-up. People in general are not particularly good takers of tablets and the elderly tend to be worse than the middle-aged and the young because of stronger objections to taking drugs and occasional forgetfulness. It is unreasonable to expect a patient to follow a complicated regime of medication which includes taking different tablets at different times of the day. The drug treatment of illness in the elderly must be as simple as possible. Drugs of doubtful therapeutic efficacy should never be used and drugs that are necessary and effective should be prescribed as simply as possible and this should be coupled with a clear explanation to the patient of what it is all about.

There used to be a custom that is now gradually dying out of prescribing most drugs three times a day. Many preparations used are long-acting and it is usually possible to reduce the frequency of dose to twice or once daily. Drugs that can be given in one dose at night are those most likely to be taken regularly and for reliability of being taken come a good second to long-acting preparations that can be given by injection by a nurse.

The drugs used commonly in psychiatry can be divided into three main groups:

Tranquillisers

Tranquillisers are preparations that it is claimed counter anxiety and agitation without producing sedation. This is in part true, but most tranquillisers if given in sufficient amounts also produce sedation and in some individuals produce considerable sedation in relatively small amounts. It is conventional to divide the tranquillisers into the major and minor variety. The latter group include medazipan (Nobrium) and diazapam (Valium). The major tranquillisers include chlorpromazine (Largactil), trifluoperazine (Stelazine), thioradazine (Melleril) and fluphenazine (Moditen).

The minor tranquillisers are normally used in the treatment of anxiety and agitation, while the major tranquillisers are used for schizophrenia, paraphrenia and other so-called psychotic reactions. This does not mean that there is a sharp division between the major and minor tranquillisers, since chlorpromazine or fluphenazine may be used to counter anxiety in neurotic reactions, while a minor tranquilliser may be used as an adjunct to treatment in the major psychoses.

There is quite a range of both minor and major tranquillisers but it is best to limit the number an individual doctor uses so that he can become familiar with their actions, side-effects and dangers. The dose ranges of the various tranquillisers are well known and it is ill-advised to lay down specific doses of drugs within this range, particularly in the elderly. Different patients respond differently to the same dose of a preparation, so rules are not possible except for one, which is that the dose should be as small as possible, compatible with producing the necessary therapeutic effect. Old people often have defects in their detoxication mechanism so that drugs build up rapidly and can produce serious side effects. Because of this the dose of any drug, be it digoxin or thioradazine, should be carefully considered and regularly reviewed. This does not mean that ridiculously small doses should be used since this is a waste of the preparation and a disservice to the patient. I have seen a very agitated old lady whose agitation was a symptom of depression being treated with 25 mg of chlorpromazine twice a day. Naturally this did not produce any improvement.

Tranquillisers can have deleterious effects on old people and often their use can be discontinued when the patient is having reasonable daily activity, including occupation and entertainment. This does not apply when the patient is a victim of a major psychosis, say paraphrenia. Here medication is important and perhaps the best method of giving it is by long-acting injection. Fluphenazine enanthate (Moditen enanthate) fluphenazine decanoate (Modecate) and fluphenthixol decanoate (Depixol) are three such preparations. Fluphenazine decanoate has now superseded the enanthate. The dose of fluphenazine decanoate is from 6.25 mg (0.25 ml) to 25 mg (1 ml) while the dose of flupenthixol decanoate is in the range 10 mg (0.5 ml) to 40 mg (2 ml). When these preparations are used a small test dose should always be tried first to ascertain if side effects are likely to occur. The side effects are usually extrapyramidal symptoms which, if severe, can be extremely distressing and even hazardous. Some psychiatrists would automatically give an anti-Parkinsonism drug such as benzhexol (Artane), orphenadrine hydrochloride (Disipal) or procyclidine (Kenadrin) when treating a patient with the long-acting phenothiazines or when giving any major tranquilliser by mouth. Others oppose this regime, claiming it is a manifestation of poly-pharmacy. They would either advocate the use of anti-Parkinson drugs only when side effects occur, or not even then, preferring to reduce the dose of tranquilliser. The long-acting preparations referred to are given at two to four weekly intervals, the interval depending of course on the patient's response to treatment.

Haloperidol (Serenace) is a useful tranquilliser for anxiety, mania and hypomania. This preparation can be given in doses of from 0.75 mg to 5 mg twice daily, or higher if necessary. It can produce extra pyramidal symptoms which are again either treated with an anti-Parkinsonism drug or by reducing the amount of haloperidol given.

Sedatives and Hypnotics

Of all the drugs at present in use, sedatives and hypnotics are possibly the most over-prescribed and ill-advisedly used. In spite of warnings, exhortations and demonstrations of their potential dangers, too many people still receive too many sedatives.

Barbiturates and Mandrax are the most abused and carry the greatest dangers. There is much publicity about young drug addicts who take amphetamines, use cannabis or LSD and sometimes become hooked on the opiates. The much larger group of middle-aged people dependent on barbiturates is rarely mentioned, yet dependence on a barbiturate can be much more damaging than smoking cannabis occasionally or taking amphetamines at a party.

There is no reason to prescribe a barbiturate as a sedative and the only barbiturates that need to be used are the short-acting ones used in anaesthesia, and phenobarbitone which may still have a place in the treatment of epilepsy. Barbiturates certainly should never be prescribed for the elderly patient, not because of the danger of dependence but due to the serious ill effects they may have upon the patient. Many old people become muddled and confused when given barbiturates and this is sometimes associated with increased restlessness and giddiness so that they may get out of bed in a muddled state and injure themselves. Some patients develop a full-blown toxic confusion, while others awake in the morning semi-drugged and depressed. Mandrax can be equally dangerous.

If an old person complains of sleeplessness it is important first to discover the true state of affairs and then if necessary try simple remedies. Many old people go to bed remarkably early for a variety of reasons, including boredom and poverty. Going to bed early can save on fuel bills. If they go to bed early they are liable to wake up very early in the morning and either complain of this or relatives become anxious. Treatment is not the giving of a sedative since it is usually possible to solve the problems which make old people go to bed early, and this in turn results in their sleeping during the normal hours.

A hot drink, a bed made more comfortable and perhaps an alcoholic nightcap can solve a number of other sleep problems in the elderly. If the patient suffers from a depressive illness, treatment of the depression can by itself correct the associated sleep disturbance.

The antidepressant amitriptyline has some sedative action and one dose, which may range from 25 to 100 mg, given last thing at night can result in the patient having a good night's sleep and also reaping the benefits of the antidepressant action, without having to worry either about taking the drug during the day, or being troubled by sleepiness.

If there is a definite need for a night sedative, dichloralphenazone (Welldorm) or trichloral are relatively safe and effective. Nitrazepam (Mogodon) is useful provided it is not used over a prolonged period, since there is evidence that it might produce confusion after long use.

The availability of a variety of tranquillisers makes the use of sedatives during the day quite unnecessary. The rule with sedatives in the elderly is the same as with any drug for this age group: only use a drug if really necessary, then use it in the smallest dose compatible with producing the required result.

Antidepressants

There are now a large number of antidepressants on the market, but there are only three main groups, the monoamineoxidase inhibitors, the tricyclics and the quadracyclics. Examples of the first group are phenelzine (Nardil), isocarboxazid (Marplan) and tranylcypromine (Parnate). Examples of tricyclics are amitriptyline (Tryptizol, Laroxyl, Saroten, and its long-acting form Lentizol), nortriptyline (Aventyl), protriptyline (Concordin) imipramine (Tofranil) and disipramine (Pertofran). The quadracyclics have only been recently introduced, and one example of this group is mianserin hydrochloride (Bolvidon, Norval).

Opinions differ about the use of monoamineoxidase inhibitors, but some psychiatrists consider that they are particularly effective in the treatment of so-called neurotic depression, while the tricyclics are more effective in the treatment of endogenous or psychotic depression. The disadvantage of using monoamineoxidase inhibitors is that they cannot be given at the same time as a whole range of other drugs, including adrenalin, the amphetamines, ephedrine, tricyclic antidepressants, narcotics, analgesics, anti-Parkinsonism drugs, sympathetic neurone blockers, ganglion blockers and thiazides and similar oral diuretics. Certain foods which contain amines or amine precursors such as cheese, Bovril, Marmite and young broad beans with pods cannot be eaten by patients taking a monoamineoxidase inhibitor. Because of these prohibitions many elderly patients cannot be given monoamineoxidase inhibitors in case they may need the incompatible drugs in an emergency in the future, or they may transgress as far as their eating habits are concerned. This does not mean that monoamineoxidase inhibitors can never be used, but the number of patients who can be treated with them is rather limited. One important factor is the ability and desire of the patient to observe carefully the prohibitions or be in a situation in which someone else can ensure this observation.

The most commonly used antidepressant is amitriptyline or its sustained release variant, Lentizol. Many people with depression are also agitated and it used to be conventional to give both an antidepressant and a tranquilliser. It is rarely necessary to do this with amitriptyline since it has tranquillising properties. If the patient is particularly withdrawn and anergic protriptyline (Concordin) may be the antidepressant of choice, while for the patient in whom amitriptyline produces too much sedation, yet there is an element of agitation, nortriptyline (Aventyl) can be very useful. The normal dose range of amitriptyline and nortriptyline is 25–50 mg twice daily and proptriptyline 10–20 mg twice daily. The dose of Lentizol is from 50—100 mg at night. If one preparation in a reasonable dose is not working it is better to change to another preparation rather than push up the amount to possibly toxic levels. The dose range for mianserin hydrochloride (Bolvidon, Norval) is from 10–20 mg twice to three times a day.

Some years ago lithium carbonate (Camcolit) was introduced as a treatment for mania. There is good evidence that this preparation can be effective in the treatment of depression and there is also evidence that it can be a fairly effective prophylactic agent to prevent recurrent attacks. Lithium carbonate is effective within fairly narrow blood levels, below which it is ineffective and above which it may produce serious toxic effects. Because of this, if lithium carbonate is used it is essential that blood levels are regularly monitored and the dose suitably altered. With this proviso there are no reasons why lithium should not be used in the treatment of the elderly.

Side effects of drugs

It has been emphasised that most effective drugs have side effects, and sometimes these side effects can be extremely serious. Old people are particularly liable to develop side effects and it is important that there is a constant awareness of this if drugs are used in treatment. It is not possible in this book to describe every drug that may be used and the side effects that may result from using that drug. However, it is important that the side effects of commonly used drugs are well understood. These are laid out in Table 1.

Effective drugs always have dangers associated with their use and it is important to discover what these may be before the drug is used. It is also important to weigh up the possible good effects of the drugs against the possible dangers. When this is done it may be decided that it is better not to use the drug than expose the patient to whatever risks there are of side effects.

Old people often receive a variety of drugs for a variety of conditions and here it is of utmost importance that not only are

TABLE 1 Side effects of drugs commonly used in psychiatry

The side effects mentioned can but do not necessarily occur, and few people would experience many of these. Mild side effects are fairly common but serious ones are rare.

Official name	*Trade name*	*Minor side effects*	*Serious side effects*
MAJOR TRANQUILLISERS			
Chlorpromazine hydrochloride	Largactil	Drowsiness Dry mouth Nasal stuffiness Drop in blood pressure Rashes Photosensitivity Weight increase Lactation	Jaundice (due to effect on liver) Leucocytosis or Leucopenia Agranulocytosis Extrapyramidal symptoms Impotence
Thioridazine	Melleril	Drowsiness Dizziness Dry mouth Lactation Nasal stuffiness Weight gain	Impotence
Perphenazine	Fentazin	Drowsiness Dry mouth	Extrapyramidal symptoms
Promazine hydrochloride	Sparine	Drowsiness Drop in blood pressure Skin rashes	Agranulocytosis
Trifluoperazine	Stelazine	Lassitude Drowsiness Dizziness Insomnia Dry mouth Blurring of vision Muscular weakness Drop in blood pressure Lactation Rashes	Extrapyramidal symptoms Jaundice (due to effect on liver) Agranulocytosis Leucopenia Thrombocytopenia

Official name	*Trade name*	*Minor side effects*	*Serious side effects*
Haloperidol	Serance		Extrapyramidal symptoms
Fluphenazine Flupenthixol	Modicate Depixol (these can be given orally or as an injection, with a prolonged action)	Drowsiness Lethargy Blurred vision Dry mouth Drop in blood pressure Lactation Skin rashes	Extrapyramidal symptoms Jaundice
MINOR TRANQUILLISERS			
Diazepan	Valium	Drowsiness	Ataxia
Chlordiazepoxide hydrochloride	Librium	Drowsiness	Ataxia
ANTIDEPRESSANTS (TRICYCLICS)			
Amitriptyline	Tryptizol Saroten Domical Lentizol	Drop in blood pressure Palpitations Drowsinesss Blurred vision Skin rashes Nausea, vomiting, giddiness Unsteady gait Lactation	Myocardial infarction Agranulocytosis Leucopenia Eosinophilia Thrombocytopenia Decreased libido Impotence
Protiptyline hydrochloride	Concordin	see amitriptyline	see amitriptyline
Nortriptyline hydrochloride	Aventyl		see amitriptyline
Imipramine hydrochloride	Tofranil	Dry mouth Increasing heart rate Difficulty in focussing eyes Constipation Sweating, giddiness Skin rashes	Disturbance of sexual functions

Official name	*Trade name*	*Minor side effects*	*Serious side effects*
ANTIDEPRESSANTS (TETRACYCLICS)			
Mianserin hydhochloride	Bolvidon Norval	Drowsiness	NOTE Both tricyclic and tetracyclic antidepressants can have ill effects on patients with glaucoma, urinary retention, pyloric stenosis and prostatic hypertrophy
ANTIDEPRESSANTS (MONOAMINEOXIDASE INHIBITORS)			
Phenelzine	Nardil	Dizziness Drowsiness Weakness Fatigue Dryness of mouth Constipation	Sexual disturbances including impotence Cerebral haemorrhage can occur
Tranylcypromine sulphate	Parnate	Headache Muscle twitching Sweating Blurring of vision Skin rashes Insomnia	Sexual disturbances including impotence Cerebral haemorrhage can occur
Lithium carbonate	Camcolit	Nausea Loose stools Fine tremor of the hands Polyuria Polydipsia Weight gain Oedema	Coarse tremor of the hands Sluggishness Sleepiness Vertigo Dysarthria Hypothyroidism
SEDATIVES			
Barbiturates		DO NOT USE	
Nitrazepan	Mogadon	Morning drowsiness	sub-acute toxic confusion after prolonged use

Official name	*Trade name*	*Minor side effects*	*Serious side effects*
Triclofos sodium	Trichloryl	Rashes Mild headache Gastro intestinal disturbances	
RIGIDITY AND TREMOR CONTROLLERS			
Benzhexol hydrochloride	Artane	Dryness of mouth Blurring of vision Dizziness Mild nausea	Acute and sub-acute toxic confusion
Orphenadrine hydrochloride	Disipal	Dryness of mouth Blurring of vision	Retention of urine
Procyclidine hydrochloride	Kemadrin	Dryness of mouth Blurring of vision Giddiness	NOTE All these preparations may have adverse effects on glaucoma and precipitate retention of urine in cases of prostatic hypertrophy

the side effects of these drugs well understood, but the danger of interaction between various drugs is also understood. Patients are often aware that certain drugs 'do not suit them', and it is unbelievably arrogant on the part of the doctor to disregard these views. One old lady said that she was always upset by imipramine but in spite of this she was persuaded to take this drug, and as a consequence became quite ill, with vomiting, tachycardia, giddiness and a skin rash.

In this chapter I have tried to describe briefly the sort of treatments that are available to old people with psychiatric illness. Further details of these treatments are available in standard works on psychiatry and monographs on specific facets of treatment. The importance of a global approach to treatment has been emphasised and, if this approach is used, very many elderly patients will be helped who otherwise may have been looked upon as beyond the help of modern medicine.

Russell Barton published his book *Institutional Neurosis* in 1966. Latterly it has been claimed that what was said in this book is now rather out of date and that the methods he suggested for combating institutional neurosis have not only become generally accepted but considerably improved upon. This is hardly the case, since a visit to many psychiatric hospitals and units and geriatric departments will reveal large numbers of patients sitting around doing nothing and never likely to do anything. A careful study of *Institutional Neurosis* and an attempt to implement the suggestions made would result in these wards of hopeless people being converted into active therapeutic communities from which many patients would be able to leave and re-establish themselves in the community.

CHAPTER 12

Conclusions

THIS BOOK is an attempt to show what can be done to help old people with mental illness. Various treatments have been described, but treatment in the narrow sense is not all-important. Little is really understood in the scientific sense about mental disorders and it may be that the various specific treatments, particularly drug therapy and other physical approaches, are based on serious misconceptions. It is important in psychiatry to be aware that we do not know, and hence to retain an open mind, so that we are not trapped into believing that this or that is *the* treatment and that it must be given even against the wishes of the patient. The important thing when treating old people is firstly and always to remember that they are people and treat them as such. Secondly, every effort should be made to provide them with help and relief, provided this help and relief is acceptable to them and is not harmful.

The treatment of patients with dementia is a good example of what can be done without having to rely on some specific treatment. There is no specific treatment for dementia, but most victims of this illness can be helped and supported so that they can end their lives relatively free of misery. It may be claimed that reality gives the lie to these claims: geriatric wards and psychiatric hospitals are gradually filling up with elderly patients, the majority of whom are labelled as suffering from dementia, with or without other diseases, and these patients linger on, becoming progressively more and more incapable of doing anything. This is certainly true but should not mean that it is inevitable. If it is accepted that certain symptoms occurring in old people, such as memory defects, confusion, incontinence, a tendency to wander and get lost, emotional lability, failure to carry out simple everyday tasks etc., indicate the existence of a disease which is untreatable and progressive, little will be done to help them and those responsible for their care will, consciously or unconsciously, assist them into the role of total dependence. This, in turn, will convince staff that their original expectations were correct, so the process will be repeated again and again. Study of the case notes of elderly patients in any psychiatric hospital will reveal, without the need of any other investigations, that this attitude is dangerous. Every hospital has some patients who were diagnosed as being demented, with the diagnosis confirmed by their subsequent behaviour, with such descriptions in their notes as "this old lady is now completely out of touch and is incapable of doing anything for herself. She is doubly incontinent, requires full nursing care, including feeding and is sometimes restless and noisy". Yet, subsequent notes will paint a very different picture: she will be described as actively busying herself in the ward, going to the canteen unattended and involving herself in social activities, including visits to the local town. This kind of history suggests that either the original diagnosis of dementia was incorrect or the dementing process can be reversed. The more popular view of these cases is that there had been a mistake in diagnosis. Provided the term 'dementia' is only applied to patients in whom there is irrefutable evidence of progressive brain destruction, this view is possibly correct. Unfortunately, we must usually make a diagnosis of dementia, if we have to, on clinical evidence, since special investigations tend to be either unreliable or potentially dangerous. For example, electroencephalography and brain scans can be misleading, while air studies which can at times fairly firmly confirm the diagnosis do place the patient at risk of unpleasant complications. Since the diagnosis must often be made on clinical grounds alone, there is always the danger of it being incorrect. Even when the diagnosis is correct, the fact that a label of dementia has been attached to a patient, can result in very little being done to help him make the most of his remaining abilities. For these two reasons alone, it is important that people who are involved in the treatment and care of the elderly should not have attitudes which encompass the belief that it is a waste of time trying to do anything for the demented.

Another consequence of the hopeless attitude to dementia is that elderly patients, not initially labelled as demented may be admitted into a ward or treated by a service that encourages demented behaviour. A patient may suffer from a straightforward easy-to-diagnose depression and, because of fears of suicide, social difficulties or other reasons, is admitted to hospital for treatment. The treatment may consist of antidepressants or ECT which should result in the patient getting better. Unfortunately, if the treatment service has an aura of pessimism as far as the elderly are concerned, a number of things may happen which will work against any beneficial effects of the simple antidepressant treatment and can result in the patient becoming apparently demented, being so labelled and never leaving hospital again. In the first place, the decision to admit may have been ill-advised with the patient becoming very upset on entering hospital and failing to come to terms with the institution.

Whether or not the admission is ill-advised, the hospital may pursue a rigid, authoritarian keep-trouble-away-at-all-costs regime in which the patient is expected to do everything she is told to do, is not allowed to make any decision or to use her initiative and is exposed to the dangers of almost total inactivity.

In the past, elderly patients were put to bed on admission and stayed there until finally they died, having become bundled up little skeletons with their chins resting on their knees. This does not happen now, but the fact that patients sit out of bed, often under the restraint of the geriatric chair, does not necessarily make the situation any better. No say, no occupation, no purpose, no conversation and no hope for the future can quickly destroy the personality of many younger people – the destructiveness in the elderly is much greater. It should not be surprising that patients exposed to this sort of regime quickly come to behave as if they were demented. Memory appears to be impaired, initiative is lost, reasoning abilities atrophy, incontinence is forced upon them and withdrawal becomes a refuge from the miseries of reality,

One method of preventing the destructive effects of the institution on old people is to develop services that make admission to the institution unnecessary. This is obviously insufficient in itself, since services that support old people in the community can be almost as destructive as some institutional services, and a proportion of old people will continue to need some form of supervised residential care. The need to treat and support as many patients in the community as possible is obvious, but this philosophy must also be combined with the development of a service whose personnel are optimistic, encouraging and view old people, even when they appear to be severely demented, as individuals who have a past and a future, have needs, desires, opinions, thoughts and the right occasionally to be difficult, unco-operative and self willed. The prevalence of this attitude will ensure that patients who are treated in the community are helped and not damaged and make institutional care for those that need it a very good second-best to successful support in the community.

The development and maintenance of the attitudes described may be looked upon as an impossible ideal. It may be said that a few people may have these attitudes but not the majority, so that any attempt to develop a hopeful, therapeutically effective service is doomed at the outset because of shortages of appropriately motivated personnel. This pessimistic view is incorrect since any group of people, be it staff of a hospital, old people's home or community service, are considerably influenced by the ethos and general atmosphere of the institutions or service team. If the group is large enough there will be a reasonably normal distribution of attitudes, with some tending towards the extreme of hopefulness and respect for the individual, and others tending towards the opposite. The majority will be somewhere in the middle. If the philosophy and atmosphere of the institution tends towards one extreme or the other the majority in the middle will tend to deviate in the same direction. In an institution where cruelty is accepted very many people will behave in a cruel manner, while a similar group of people in a kindly institution will tend to have a high incidence of kindness.

The development of the philosophy and atmosphere is dependent upon the people in charge of the service or, if it is run on more democratic lines, those members who have been elected to positions of administrative responsibility.

Remembering the importance of attitude, the type of service that should be developed and evolved can be considered.

Future developments

It was pointed out in Chapter 4 (Facilities and the Psychiatric Team) that in spite of obvious disadvantages, it does appear essential that special units should be established for the treatment and care of elderly people with mental illness. Many such units already exist but their number will remain inadequate until every area in the country is served by them. In the first place, a large proportion of these units will be based on psychiatric hospitals because it is here that so many old people are incarcerated. Since there are large numbers of old people in psychiatric hospitals, it is essential that the special units are developed there so that they, as well as the old in the community who become ill, receive the type of treatment and support to which they are entitled. There is an unfortunate tendency to develop new and progressive psychiatric services that exclude the mental hospital population of long-stay patients. These unfortunates having failed to benefit from the advances in psychiatry that have occurred, either because they were admitted there too long ago or for other reasons including rejection by over-pessimistic psychiatrists, now tend to be forgotten and so continue unhelped by these advances. It does appear that the movement towards general hospital and community psychiatry is possibly best for both patient and society, but this movement should not occur at the expense of those that society has neglected for so long. Because of this it is important that psychiatric hospitals should continue to serve active functions until they are finally emptied of patients, closed and demolished. The development of active,

psychogeriatric units in the psychiatric hospital is one of many ways of ensuring an active, progressive atmosphere until final closure.

When a unit for the elderly is established it is important that a day hospital and a service to patients in the community should be a integral part of that unit. Following the creation of this community-orientated unit, the next stage is to devise plans for its total removal from the psychiatric hospital to the general hospital and community milieu. This can be done in a number of ways, including the total removal of the unit to the general hospital or the removal of the acute work there with the provision of longer stay accommodation in community hospitals, hostels, housing projects etc. If the latter course is accepted the whole complex of facilities should still remain an integral part of the unit under the same direction and with a free flow of staff between the different facilities.

During the early stages of the development of a unit, real efforts must be made to forge close and effective links with other services for the elderly. Important services with whom there should be close links include the geriatric service, local authority facilities for the elderly, the family doctor service and the fairly large range of voluntary bodies involved in providing help for the old. It is very popular to talk about liaison and co-operation, but too often this means the establishment of some multi-disciplinary committee the members of which meet and drearily discuss mutual problems and possible solutions without ever really becoming involved personally in the problems of patients and the morass of services intended to help them, frequently being more interested in ensuring that the problem does not become theirs. There is a game which has been christened 'geriatric pass-the-parcel' that can be played between different departments. In this game the old person is the parcel and the object of the exercise is to keep passing her until she finally ends up with one agency who is looked upon as the loser. Liaison committees frequently perpetuate the game by laying down rules when, in fact, their function should be to make it unplayable. True liaison and co-operation can only occur at the working level: this means that the administration of the various organisations should be designed to encourage and allow close working relationships between workers in different services and the creation of an atmosphere in which all workers look upon problems as everyone's concern.

A case can be made out for the total integration of psychiatric services for the elderly into the geriatric service and this may be the best development. However, there is room for experimentation so it is possibly best that different areas develop different methods of co-ordinating services which later can be compared, with the object of using the best in each organisation as a composite model for the future. There is a clearly demonstrable danger in creating inflexible organisations, examples of which are always before our eyes. A well-constructed organisation that works but is inflexible is a very dangerous organisation. Situations are always changing and an inflexible organisation cannot deal with change. If it is badly organised it will collapse under the stress of change, but if it is well organised it might survive to the organisation's advantage but not to the advantage of anyone else.

The possibility of the total integration of geriatric and psychiatric services for the elderly is often discussed but a truly integrated and comprehensive service must include very close relationships with many other services and organisations. These include the usual local authority and voluntary services but must also encompass other branches of medicine and surgery. Medicine in general is becoming more and more the diagnosis, treatment and support of old people. Many medical and surgical wards have almost as many elderly patients as a so-called geriatric or psychogeriatric ward. In spite of this development, a surprising number of physicians and surgeons appear to live in a fantasy world in which all their patients are young and are, to use their term, curable, while old people who may not be so curable are looked upon as a nuisance that should be quickly got rid of to the geriatrician or psychiatrist. This attitude not only causes tension within the medical services but tends to perpetuate the second-rate status of services specifically organised to deal with old people. The answer to this problem must lie with medical, nursing and administrative education.

Education

Every developed society has an increasing proportion of elderly people, which should mean that these societies ought to study their educational systems with a view to modifying them to deal with this phenomenon. Changes in education should encompass the general public, so that they are better able to deal with old age in themselves and in others, and the professionals so that they are prepared to deal with old people effectively in their day-to-day practice.

The treatment and care of old people can be a rewarding and satisfying experience which is often superior to that achieved when dealing with other age groups. Past situations, uniformed preconceptions and unfortunate attitudes in older professionals are some of the causes of geriatric medicine and psychiatry being so unpopular at the present time. These attitudes must be changed and can be changed provided those responsible for education are aware of the problem and have any interest at all in providing a solution.

The need for a more democratic approach

Medicine and nursing is traditionally autocratic and most medical services are developed and run with little regard for the views of the public or the patients. In countries which lack a health service, doctors work in ways that have little regard for what the public think or want. A National Health Service such as that provided in the United Kingdom is also something that has been developed and functions remote from the public's will. Following its recent re-organisation, Community Health Councils were established which unfortunately have little power, but perhaps their power will be increased.

Health and social services should be developed along lines that satisfy the needs and desires of the whole of society. There should be much more involvement of the public and patients in all levels of administration so that genuine attempts may be made to produce services that satisfy the public need. The introduction of democracy into the health and social services would not lead, as many claim, to the professional being ignored but would mean that he would have to give cogent reasons for his decisions instead of the present situation in which he expresses his opinion as if it were an irrefutable truth. Public participation in health and welfare services would mean more than simply making democracy more of a reality. It would make the professional think much more about what he was doing, broaden his horizons and tap a wealth of knowledge and understanding that is at present hidden outside the walls of professionalism.

There is an urgent need to explore ways in which the powers and involvement of Community Health Councils can be enlarged, so that they provide a genuine opportunity for the public to influence what goes on within the Health Service, at the same time extending this function to Local Authority provisions, such as Social Service Departments, Housing Departments etc.

Mental illness in the elderly will continue to be a problem to our society until it is realised that humane solutions are available provided we have the interest and concern to use them.

Bibliography

General reading

Bromley D. (1966) *The Psychology of Human Ageing*. London: Penguin Books.

Comfort A. (1965) *The Process of Ageing*. London: Weidenfeld & Nicholson.

Goffman E. (1961) *Asylums*. Anchor.

Revans R. W. (1966) *Standards for Moral Cause and Effects in Hospitalisation*. Oxford University Press.

Robb B. *Sans Everything*. London: Nelson.

Roberts N. *Our Future Selves*. London: Allen & Unwin.

Psychiatry

Barton R. (1966) *Institutional Neurosis*. Bristol: Wright.

Gostin L. O. (1977) *A Human Condition*. MIND (NAMH).

Grossman K. Granville (1976) *Recent Advances in Clinical Psychiatry*. Churchill Livingstone.

Mayer-Gross W., Slater E. & Roth M. (1969) *Clinical Psychiatry*. London: Baillière, Tindall.

Sainsbury M. J. (1976) *Key to Psychiatry*. Aylesbury: HM+M Publishers.

The Mental Health Act 1959. HMSO.

Geriatric medicine

Agate J. M. (1970) *The Practice of Geriatrics*. London: Heinemann.

Anderson W. F. (1071) *Practical Management of the Elderly*. Oxford: Blackwell.

Felstein I. (1969) *Later Life – Geriatrics Today and Tomorrow*. London: Penguin Books.

Hall M. R. P., MacLennan W. J. & Lye M. D. W. (1978) *Medical Care of the Elderly*. Aylesbury: HM+M Publishers.

Hazell K. (1973) *Social and Medical Problems of the Elderly*. London: Hutchinson.

Howell T. H. (1970) *A Student's Guide to Geriatrics*. London: Staples Press.

Hyams D. (1973) *Care of the Aged*. London: Priory Press.

Irving R. E., Bagnall M. K. & Smith B. J. (1968) *The Older Patient: an Introduction to Geriatrics*. London: English University Press.

Isaacs B. (Editor) (1978) *Recent Advances in Geriatric Medicine*. Edinburgh: Churchill-Livingstone.

Stewart M. C. (1970) *My Brother's Keeper.* London: Health Horizon.

Mental illness in the elderly

Bergmann K. (1973) *The Aged – Their Understanding and Care.* London: Wolfe Publishing.

Corsellis J. A. N. (1962) *Mental Illness and the Ageing Brain.* Oxford University Press.

Pitt Brice (1976) *Psychogeriatrics.* Edinburgh: Churchill-Livingstone.

Social aspects

Fry M. *Old Age in the Modern World.* Edinburgh: Churchill-Livingstone.

Hall M. P. (1971) *The Social Services of Modern England.* London: Routledge & Kegan Paul.

Meacher M. (1972) *Taken for a Ride.* Longman.

Rudd T. N. (1967) *Human Relations in Old Age.* London: Faber.

Townsend P. (1970) *The Family Life of Old People.* London: Penguin Books.

Townsend P. (1964) *The Last Refuge.* London: Routledge & Kegan Paul.

Nursing

Adams G. F. & McIlwraith (1963) *Geriatric Nursing.* Oxford University Press.

Exton-Smith A. N. (1955) *Medical Problems of Old Age.* Bristol: Wright.

McLeod F. (1976) *Geriatric Care (Nursing Modules Series).* Aylesbury: HM+M Publishers.

Rudd T. N. (1964) *The Nursing of the Elderly Sick.* London: Faber.

Services

Whitehead T. (1978) *In the Service of Old Age.* Aylesbury: HM+M Publishers.

Neurology

Brain, Lord Russell (1973) *Clinical Neurology.* Oxford University Press.

Walshe, Sir Francis (1970) *Diseases of the Nervous System.* Edinburgh: Churchill-Livingstone.

Index